Air Fryer Cookbook

500 Quick and Delicious Recipes for Beginners and Advanced Users

(+ Out Of The Box Tips & Tricks)

BY
Linda Vogel

Table of Contents

Introduction

Congratulations on purchasing your personal copy of the *Air Fryer Cookbook* and thank you for doing so. I will explain how to use an Air Fryer for a complete beginner from start to finish. The Air Fryer is capable of functioning like so many products, whether you need an oven, a hot grill, a toaster, a skillet, or a deep fryer—it is your answer! It can be used for breakfast, lunch, dinner, desserts, and even snacks.

The compact air fryer allows you to set the cooking temperature and timer. All you need to do is wait for the beep, and your food is ready for the table. You won't have a messy workspace since there isn't much to clean. Cooking food in the fryer is fast, safe, and healthy – anytime - day or night.

The machine will automatically shut down when the cooking time is completed. You will have less burned or overheated food items. The fryer will not slip because of the non-slip feet which help eliminate the risk of the machine from falling off of the countertop. The closed cooking system helps prevent burns from hot oil or other foods.

Let's get started!

Chapter 1: Breakfast Egg Favorites

Asparagus Omelet

Yields Provided: 2 Servings
Ingredients:
- Warm water (2 tbsp.)
- Black pepper and salt (1 pinch of each)
- Parmesan cheese (1 tbsp.)
- Eggs (3)
- Steamed asparagus tips (5)
- Spritz of cooking oil spray (as needed)

Preparation Technique:
1. Set the Air Fryer temperature at 320° Fahrenheit.
2. Whisk the water, pepper, salt, eggs, and cheese.
3. Spritz a skillet using cooking spray and steam the asparagus. Add to the fryer basket. Pour in the egg mixture.
4. Air fry for five minutes and serve.

Avocado Egg Boats

Yields Provided: 2 Servings
Ingredients:
- Avocado (1)
- Large eggs (2)
- Toppings As Desired:
  - Freshly chopped chives
  - Parsley
  - Pepper
  - Salt

Preparation Technique:
1. Warm up the fryer to 350° Fahrenheit.
2. Remove the pit from the avocado. Slice and scoop out part of the flesh. Shake with the seasonings.
3. Add an egg to each half and place it in the Air Fryer. Set the timer for six minutes.
4. Serve using the toppings of your preference.

Baked Eggs In A Bread Bowl

Yields Provided: 4 egg bowls
Ingredients:
- Large eggs (4)
- Crusty dinner rolls (4)
- Heavy cream (4 tbsp.)
- Mixed herbs - ex. Chopped tarragon, chives, parsley, etc. (4 tbsp. ea.)
- Grated parmesan cheese (to your liking)

Preparation Technique:
1. Set the Air Fryer at 350° Fahrenheit.
2. Use a sharp knife to remove the top of each of the rolls – setting them aside for later. Scoop out some of the bread to form a hole large enough for the egg.
3. Place the rolls in the fryer basket. Break an egg into the roll and top with the cream and herbs. Sprinkle using a portion of the parmesan.
4. Bake for about 20 to 25 minutes until the egg is set. The bread should be toasted.
5. After 20 minutes, arrange the tops of the bread on the egg and bake a few more minutes to finish the browning process.
6. Remove from the Air Fryer and wait for five minutes. Serve warm.

Barbecued Eggs

Yields Provided: 4 Servings
Ingredients - For the Sauce:
- Ketchup (1 cup)
- Apple cider vinegar (.25 cup)
- Brown sugar (2 tbsp.)
- Onion powder (.5 tsp.)
- Mustard powder (.5 tsp.)
- Molasses (2 tbsp.)
- Worcestershire sauce (1 tbsp.)
- Liquid smoke (.5 tsp.)

Ingredients:
- Eggs (4)
- Bacon (12 slices)
- Pepper and salt (to your liking)
- Butter (1 tbsp.)
- Sliced croissants (2)
- Softened butter (4 tbsp.)

Preparation Technique:
1. Set the Air Fryer temperature to 390° Fahrenheit.
2. Using the medium-heat temperature setting on the stovetop, mix the brown sugar, vinegar, molasses, ketchup, onion powder, and mustard powder in a small pan.
3. Whisk the liquid smoke and Worcestershire sauce into the mixture to blend thoroughly. Cook until the sauce thickens. Add additional flavoring as desired.
4. Arrange the bacon on the trays and fry for five minutes. Remove and brush the bacon with the barbecue sauce – flip – and brush the other side. Arrange it back in the cooker, and cook for another five minutes.
5. Butter a halved croissant, and toast it in the fryer.
6. In the meantime, use a non-stick pan on the med-low setting on the stovetop to melt the butter. Add four

eggs to the pan, cooking until the white starts setting. Flip and cook about thirty more seconds.

7. Serve with the bacon and croissant.

Biscuit Bombs

Yields Provided: 10 Servings
Ingredients:
- Vegetable oil (1 tbsp.)
- Bulk breakfast sausage (.25 lb.)
- Eggs (2)
- Salt & pepper (.125 tsp.)
- Pillsbury Grands - Flaky Layers (5-count)
- Sharp cheddar cheese (2 oz.)
- For the Egg Wash (1 tbsp. water + 1 egg)
- *Also Needed*: 10-inch skillet

Preparation Technique:
1. Use a sheet of parchment baking paper to prepare two 8-inch rounds. Fit one of the pieces in the bottom of the Air Fryer basket. Spritz using a cooking oil spray.
2. Warm the vegetable oil in a frying pan using the med-high temperature setting.
3. Toss in the sausage to cook until the pink is gone (2-5 min). Place the sausage into a bowl, leaving the grease in the skillet.
4. Lower the temperature setting to medium. Whisk and add the eggs, pepper, and salt. Cook until they're thickened, but still moist. Toss the eggs into the sausage bowl to cool for 5 minutes.
5. In the meantime, divide the five biscuits; then, separate each biscuit into two layers. Press each segment into four-inch rounds.
6. Scoop one heaping tablespoonful of the egg mixture and cheese to each round. Fold the edges up and over the filling; pinching to seal.
7. Prepare the egg wash using the mixture of water and the last egg. Brush the biscuits using the egg wash.
8. Place five of the biscuit bombs into the Air Fryer basket. Use a spritz of oil to spray both sides of the second

parchment round with cooking oil spray. and arrange on the bombs in the basket with a second parchment round, then top with the five biscuit bombs.

9. Sere when ready.

Breakfast Burrito

Yields Provided: 1-2 Servings
Ingredients:
- Eggs (2)
- Chicken or turkey breast (3-4 slices)
- Avocado (.25 of 1)
- Bell pepper (.25 of 1)
- Mozzarella cheese – (.125 cup - grated)
- Pepper and salt (1 pinch each)
- Salsa (2 tbsp.)
- Tortilla (1)

Preparation Technique:
1. Slice the bell pepper and avocado; and set aside. In a small mixing container, whisk the eggs, pepper, and salt.
2. Fold the fixings into a small pan and arrange it in the Air Fryer basket.
3. Set the timer for five minutes at 392°Fahrenheit.
4. When done, transfer the egg from the pan and fill the tortilla. Combine all of the fixings and wrap it.
5. Add a piece of foil to the Air Fryer tray and add the burrito. Heat for three minutes at 356° Fahrenheit.
6. The cheese will be melted, and the tortilla crispy. Garnish as desired and serve.

Cheesy Ham – Egg & Mushroom Croissant

Yields Provided: 1 Serving
Ingredients:
- Egg (1)
- Mozzarella or cheddar cheese (1.8 oz.)
- Honey shaved ham (3 slices)
- Croissant (1)
- Halved cherry tomatoes (4)
- Small quartered button mushrooms (4)
- *Optional*: Roughly chopped rosemary sprig (.5 of 1)

Preparation Technique:
1. Help prevent the batter from sticking by lightly greasing the baking dish.
2. Warm the Air Fryer to reach 320° Fahrenheit.
3. Toss half of the cheese in the bottom of the dish. Leave a space in the center portion of the ham. Break and add the egg.
4. Toss the rosemary, salt, and pepper over the mixture.
5. Sprinkle with the last of the cheese.
6. Arrange in the basket and air fry for 8 minutes.
7. Air fry the croissant for about 4 minutes. Serve when the egg is set.

Egg & Bacon Cups

Yields Provided: 4 Servings
Ingredients:
- Eggs (4)
- Dried dill (.5 tsp.)
- Salt (.25 tsp.)
- Paprika (.5 tsp.)
- Bacon (6 oz.)
- Butter (1 tbsp.)
- _Also Needed_: 4 ramekins

Preparation Technique:
1. Preheat the Air Fryer to reach 360° Fahrenheit.
2. Use an electric mixer or just whisk the eggs, dried dill, salt, and paprika.
3. Cover the ramekins with butter. Slice the bacon and arrange it in each of the cups. Dump the egg mixture into the centers. Set the timer for 15 minutes.
4. Serve when ready.

Egg Cheese and Pepperoni Pizza

Yields Provided: 1 Serving
Ingredients:
- Eggs (2)
- Oregano (.5 tsp.)
- Basil (.5 tsp.)
- Shredded mozzarella cheese (2 tbsp.)
- Thinly sliced pepperoni (4 pieces)
- *Also Needed*: 1 ramekin

Preparation Technique:
1. Whisk the eggs with the basil and oregano.
2. Dump into the ramekin and top add the pepperoni and cheese.
3. Place the ramekin in the Air Fryer for three minutes and serve.

Eggs In A Zucchini Nest

Yields Provided: 4 Servings

Ingredients:

- Grated zucchini (8 oz.)
- Butter (4 tsp.)
- Sea salt (.25 tsp.)
- Paprika (.5 tsp.)
- Black pepper (.5 tsp.)
- Eggs (4)
- Shredded cheddar cheese (4 oz.)
- *Also Needed*: 4 ramekins

Preparation Technique:

1. Preheat the Air Fryer at 356° Fahrenheit.
2. Add the butter to the ramekins. Grate the zucchini and arrange it in the ramekins in a nest shape. Sprinkle using the salt, paprika, and pepper.
3. Briskly whisk the eggs and add to the nest, with a dusting of cheese.
4. Air fry for 7 minutes. Cool slightly for 3 minutes and serve in the ramekin.

Herbal Hard-Boiled Eggs

Yields Provided: 2 Servings
Ingredients:
- Hard-boiled eggs (4)
- Dried parsley (1 tsp.)
- Chopped chives (1 tbsp.)
- Paprika (1 tsp.)
- Sea salt (.5 tsp.)
- Oregano (1 tsp.)
- Cream (1 tbsp.

Preparation Technique:
1. Heat the Air Fryer to reach 320° Fahrenheit.
2. Gently place the eggs in the Air Fryer basket to simmer for 17 minutes. Transfer to a cold water bath to chill. Peel and slice into halves and set the white part aside.
3. Remove the yolks and mix them with the remainder of the ingredients.
4. Fill the egg white halves and serve.

Quick & Easy Poached Eggs

Yields Provided: 1 Serving
Ingredients:

- Boiling water (3 cups)
- Large egg (1)

Preparation Technique:

1. Pour boiling water into the Air Fryer basket.
2. Break the egg into a dish and slide it into the water. Set the basket into the fryer.
3. Set the timer for 3 minutes. When ready, scoop the poached egg into a plate using a slotted spoon.
4. Serve with a serving of toast to your liking.

Scrambled Eggs

Yields Provided: 1 Serving
Ingredients:
- Butter (for the basket)
- Eggs (2)
- Salt & black pepper (as desired)

Preparation Technique:
1. Set the Air Fryer temperature at 285° Fahrenheit for about five minutes.
2. Melt a small portion of butter, spreading it out evenly.
3. Whisk and dump the eggs and any other desired fixings such as cheese or tomatoes.
4. Open the fryer every few minutes to whisk the eggs to the desired consistency.
5. Serve with a side of toast or have a scrambled egg sandwich.

Spinach - Ham & Eggs Omelet

Yields Provided: 4 Servings
Ingredients:

- Sliced ham (7 oz.)
- Spinach (2.25 cups)
- Heavy cream (4 tsp.)
- Olive oil (1 tbsp.)
- Large eggs (4)
- Black pepper & salt (as desired)
- *Also Needed*: 4 ramekins & skillet

Preparation Technique:

1. Warm the Air Fryer ahead of baking time to reach 356° Fahrenheit. Spritz the ramekins with a misting of cooking oil spray.
2. Pour the oil into the skillet (med. heat). Toss in the spinach and sauté until it's wilted. Drain.
3. Divide the spinach and rest of the fixings in each of the ramekins.
4. Bake until set (20 min.). Serve when they are to your liking.

Thai Omelet

Yields Provided: 4 Servings

Ingredients:

- Sausage (.5 cup)
- Green onion (1)
- Fish sauce (2 tbsp.)
- Eggs (4)
- White pepper powder (2 tbsp.)
- Minced shallot (1)
- Garlic cloves (2)
- Lime juice (.5 of 1 lime)
- Fresh spinach (1 handful)
- *To Garnish*: Cilantro

Preparation Technique:

1. Warm the fryer to reach 340° Fahrenheit.
2. Finely chop the onion and sausage.
3. Warm oil in a frying pan. Whisk the eggs, pepper, and fish sauce; adding the rest of the fixings until combined.
4. Pour into the pan and place it into the Air Fryer basket to cook for 10 minutes.
5. Garnish and serve with a dusting of cilantro.

Western Omelet

Yields Provided: 4 Servings
Ingredients:
- Eggs (5)
- Cream cheese (3 tbsp.)
- Cilantro (1 tsp.)
- Oregano (1 tsp.)
- Shredded parmesan cheese (3 oz.)
- Green pepper (1)
- Yellow diced onion (1.5)
- Olive oil (1 tsp.)
- Butter (1 tsp.)
- *Also Needed*: 1 Skillet

Preparation Technique:
1. Whisk the eggs, cilantro, and oregano. Mix and add the cream cheese and parmesan.
2. Heat the Air Fryer ahead of time to reach 360° Fahrenheit.
3. Dump the eggs into the fryer basket. Set the timer for 10 minutes.
4. Chop the onions and peppers. Pour oil into a skillet using the medium heat setting. Sauté for 8 minutes.
5. When the eggs are done, serve and garnish with the sautéed vegetables.

Chapter 2: Breakfast & Brunch Options

Air Fryer Bagels

Yields Provided: 4 Servings
Ingredients:
- Self-rising flour (1 cup)
- Zero fat plain Greek yogurt (1 cup)
- Egg (1 for the egg wash)
- Desired garnishes: Sesame or poppy seeds

Preparation Technique:
1. Set the Air Fryer at 330° Fahrenheit ahead of baking time.
2. Whisk the yogurt and flour to form a tacky dough.
3. Dust a preparation surface and roll the dough into a ball; slicing it into four sections.
4. Roll each one into bagel shapes and pinch to close.
5. Prepare two at a time, brushing the tops with egg wash.
6. Set the timer for ten minutes after arranging the bagels in the cooker.
7. For the toppings; just brush with a portion of melted butter and season to your liking.

Bacon & Cheese Muffins

Yields Provided: 6 Servings
Ingredients:
- Large slices of bacon (4)
- Medium onion (1)
- Olive oil (2 tbsp.)
- Shredded cheddar cheese (1 cup)
- Parsley (1 tsp.)
- Almond flour (1.5 cups)
- Pepper and salt (as desired)
- Baking powder (2 tsp.)
- Milk (1 cup)
- Large egg (1)
- *Also Needed:* 6-count muffin tins to fit in the basket

Preparation Technique:
1. Warm the Air Fryer to reach 356° Fahrenheit.
2. Fry the ban using a spritz of oil. Toss in the onion when it's about halfway ready. Sauté and set aside when translucent. Drain on a layer of paper towels.
3. Mix in the rest of the fixings and stir well.
4. Dump the batter into six muffin tins.
5. Add to the fryer basket to cook for 20 minutes.
6. Reduce the temperature for 10 minutes (320° Fahrenheit).
7. Serve while piping hot.

Ham Hash

Yields Provided: 3 Servings
Ingredients:
- Ham (10 oz.)
- Parmesan (5 oz.)
- Onion (.5 of 1)
- Butter (1 tbsp.)
- Egg (1)
- Black pepper (1 tsp.)
- Paprika (1 tsp.)
- *Also Needed*: 3 ramekins

Preparation Technique:
1. Preheat the Air Fryer to reach 350° Fahrenheit.
2. Shred the parmesan cheese and slice the ham into small strips.
3. Peel and dice the onion. Lastly, whisk and mix in the egg, salt, pepper, and paprika. Combine all of the fixings together and add to the ramekins with a sprinkle of parmesan.
4. Place the ramekins in the Air Fryer for 10 minutes.
5. When ready, transfer to your plate, and scramble to serve.

Mushroom Onion & Cheese Frittata

Yields Provided: 2 Servings
Ingredients:
- Olive oil (1 tbsp.)
- Mushrooms (2 cups)
- Onion (1 small)
- Eggs (3)
- Grated cheese (50 g or .5 cup)
- Salt (1 pinch)
- *Also Needed*: 1 Skillet

Preparation Technique:
1. Set the Air Fryer temperature to 320° Fahrenheit.
2. Heat a skillet using the medium heat setting and pour in the oil.
3. Chop the mushrooms and onions. Toss into the pan and sauté for about five minutes before adding to the Air Fryer.
4. Whisk the eggs and salt. Dump it into the fryer with a sprinkle of cheese.
5. Set the timer for 10 minutes and remove to serve.

WW-Friendly Bagels

Yields Provided: 4 Servings
Ingredients:
- Greek yogurt (1 cup)
- Self-rising flour (1 cup)
- Egg (1)

Preparation Technique:
1. Warm the Air Fryer at 350° Fahrenheit.
2. Combine the yogurt and flour to form a ball of dough.
3. Place the ball onto a flat dry surface covered with flour.
4. Separate into 4 balls and roll into a long rope, shaping it into a bagel.
5. Whisk the egg. Coat each bagel with an egg wash and any toppings.
6. Arrange in the Air Fryer. Set the timer for ten minutes.

Sweet Breakfast Treats

Apple Dumplings

Yields Provided: 2 Servings
Ingredients:
- Raisins (2 tbsp.)
- Small apples (2)
- Brown sugar (1 tbsp.)
- Puff pastry (2 sheets)
- Melted butter (2 tbsp.)

Preparation Technique:
1. Peel and core the apples.
2. Heat the Air Fryer in advance to reach 356° Fahrenheit.
3. Combine the raisins and sugar. Place the apples on the pastry sheets and fill with the raisin mixture.
4. Fold the pastry over to cover the fixings. Place them on a piece of foil so they won't fall through the fryer. Brush them with melted butter.
5. Air fry until they're golden brown (25 min.).
6. *Note*: It's best to prepare using tiny apples.

Banana Fritters

Yields Provided: 8 Servings
Ingredients:
- Vegetable oil (3 tbsp.)
- Breadcrumbs (.75 cup)
- Corn flour (3 tbsp.)
- Ripe peeled bananas (8)
- Egg white (1)

Preparation Technique:
1. Set the temperature on the Air Fryer to reach 356° Fahrenheit.
2. Use the low-heat temperature setting to warm a skillet. Pour in the oil and toss in the breadcrumbs. Cook until golden brown.
3. Coat the bananas with the flour. Dip them into the whisked egg white, and cover with the breadcrumbs.
4. Arrange the prepared bananas in a single layer of the basket and set the timer for 8 minutes.
5. Transfer to paper towels to drain before serving.

Chocolate & Avocado Muffins

Yields Provided: 7 Servings

Ingredients:

- Apple cider vinegar (1 tsp.)
- Almond flour (1 cup)
- Baking soda (.5 tsp.)
- Stevia powder (3 scoops)
- Egg (1)
- Melted dark chocolate (1 oz.)
- Butter (4 tbsp.)
- Pitted avocado (.5 cup)

Preparation Technique:

1. Set the Air Fryer at 355° Fahrenheit.
2. Whisk the baking soda, almond flour, and the vinegar. Melt and add in the chocolate and stevia powder.
3. Whisk the egg in another bowl and add to the mixture along with the butter.
4. Peel, cube, and mash the avocado and add. Blend using a hand mixer until smooth. Pour into the muffin forms (halfway full). Cook for nine minutes.
5. Reduce the heat (340° Fahrenheit) and cook for another nine minutes.
6. Chill before serving for the best results.

French Toast Sticks

Yields Provided: 2 Servings

Ingredients:
- Eggs (2)
- *Spices*: Cinnamon - Nutmeg - Ground cloves (1 pinch each)
- Salt (1 pinch)
- Bread - your choice (4 slices)
- Soft margarine or butter (2 tbsp.)
- *Garnish:* Maple syrup
- Cooking oil spray (as needed)

Preparation Technique:
1. Heat the Air Fryer prior to the baking time to reach 356° Fahrenheit.
2. Whisk the eggs, nutmeg, cloves, and cinnamon.
3. Prepare using two batches. Spread butter on both sides of the bread and slice into strips. Dredge each piece in the egg mixture and place it in the Air Fryer.
4. After 2 minutes, pause and remove the pan. Lightly spray both sides of the bread using a portion of cooking oil spray. Return to the fryer for 4 more minutes.
5. Garnish with maple syrup, whipped cream, or a drizzle of confectioner's sugar. Serve them immediately.

Pumpkin Pie French Toast

Yields Provided: 4 Servings

Ingredients:

- Water (.25 cup)
- Large eggs (2)
- Pumpkin puree (.25 cup)
- Pumpkin pie spices (.25 tsp.)
- Butter (.25 cup)
- Low-carb bread (4 slices)

Preparation Technique:

1. Whisk the eggs with the water, pie spice, and pumpkin puree.
2. Once it's smooth, dip the bread into the mixture.
3. Warm the fryer to 340° Fahrenheit.
4. Once it's hot, set the timer for 10 minutes.
5. Serve with a portion of butter.

Scrambled Pancake Hash

Yields Provided: 7 Servings

Ingredients:

- Coconut flour (1 cup)
- Baking soda (1 tsp.)
- Salt (1 tsp.)
- Ground ginger (1 tsp.)
- Heavy cream (.25 cup)
- Apple cider vinegar (1 tbsp.)
- Egg (1)
- Butter (5 tbsp.)

Preparation Technique:

1. Heat the Air Fryer to reach 400° Fahrenheit.
2. Whisk the flour, ginger, baking soda, and salt in a mixing bowl.
3. In a separate container, combine the egg, butter, and cream. Blend well using a hand mixer. Combine each of the fixings and stir until creamy smooth.
4. Slowly dump the mixture into the Air Fryer tray.
5. Set the timer for 4 minutes. Remove and scramble the hash.
6. Place back into the fryer and continue to cook for another five minutes.
7. Serve piping hot.

Brunch Options

Bacon & Hot Dog Omelet

Yields Provided: 4 Servings
Ingredients:
- Sliced hot dogs (2)
- Small sliced onions (2)
- Eggs (2)
- Chopped bacon bits (1 slice)
- Black pepper & salt (to your liking)

Preparation Technique:
1. Set the temperature of the Air Fryer to reach 320° Fahrenheit.
2. Mix all of the ingredients well and pour them into the fryer tray.
3. Air fry for 10 minutes and serve.

Spinach Frittata

Yields Provided: 2 Servings
Ingredients:
- Red onion (1 small)
- Spinach (⅓ of 1 pkg.)
- Eggs (3)
- Black pepper & salt (as desired)
- Mozzarella cheese (as desired)

Preparation Technique:
1. Warm the Air Fryer to reach 356° Fahrenheit (at least 3 min.).
2. Add oil to a baking pan (one that fits in the fryer) for one minute. Mince and toss in the onions and cook for two to three minutes.
3. Toss in the spinach and cook three to five minutes more minutes.
4. Whisk and add the eggs, cheese, and seasonings into the pan.
5. Set the timer for 8 minutes. Adjust to your liking with the pepper and salt before serving.

Sweet Potato Hash

Yields Provided: 6 Servings
Ingredients:
- Large sweet potato (2)
- Bacon slices (2)
- Olive oil (2 tbsp.)
- Dried dill weed (1 tsp.)
- Smoked paprika (1 tbsp.)
- Sea salt & pepper (1 tsp. ea.)

Preparation Technique:
1. Warm the oven to reach 400° Fahrenheit.
2. Dice the sweet potato into small cubes and toss with the dill, salt, pepper, paprika, and olive oil. Fry the bacon until crispy and break into small pieces to garnish the hash.
3. Scoop the mixture into the hot fryer and air-fry for 12-16 minutes.
4. After 10 minutes, check and continue checking in 3-minute intervals until browned and crispy.

Tex-Mex Hash Browns

Yields Provided: 4 Servings

Ingredients:
- Potatoes (1.5 lb.)
- Olive oil (1 tbsp.)
- Small onion (1)
- Seeded jalapeno (1)
- Red bell pepper (1)
- Black pepper (as desired)
- Salt (1 pinch)
- Taco seasoning mix (.5 tsp.)
- Olive oil (.5 tsp.)
- Ground cumin (.5 tsp.)

Preparation Technique:
1. Soak the potatoes in cool water for 20 minutes.
2. Warm the Air Fryer to 320° Fahrenheit.
3. Drain the potatoes, dry them with a clean towel, and transfer to a large bowl.
4. Drizzle 1 tablespoon of oil over the potatoes and shake to coat. Toss them into the hot fryer basket. Set the timer for 18 minutes.
5. Put the peppers, onions, and jalapenos in the bowl previously used for the potatoes. Sprinkle in 1/2 teaspoon of oil, taco seasoning, ground cumin, salt, and pepper. Toss to coat.
6. Transfer the potatoes from the Air Fryer to the container with the veggie mixture. Return the empty basket to the fryer and raise the temperature to 356° Fahrenheit.
7. Quickly toss the contents of the bowl to mix the potatoes with the vegetables and seasonings. Transfer the mixture into the basket. Set the timer for 6 minutes, shake the basket, and continue cooking

until potatoes are browned and crispy (5 min.). Serve immediately.

Tofu Egg Muffins

Yields Provided: 4 Servings
Ingredients:
- Tofu (1 small chunk)
- Large eggs (3)
- Sesame oil (.25 tsp.)
- Cumin (.25 tsp.)
- Coriander - dried (.25 tsp.)
- Black pepper (.25 tsp.)
- Soy sauce (.5 tsp.)
- Spring onion (1 handful)
- Fresh coriander (1 handful)
- *Also Needed:* Muffin molds (4)

Preparation Technique:
1. Warm the Air Fryer at 392° Fahrenheit for about five minutes.
2. Combine all of the fixings except for the tofu, whisking well. Break the tofu into equal portions in the mold and add the mixture over each one.
3. Arrange the muffins in the Air Fryer and air-fry for ten minutes.

Chapter 3: Lunch Specialties

Chicken Hash

Yields Provided: 3 Servings
Ingredients
- Chicken fillet (7 oz.)
- Cauliflower (6 oz.)
- Yellow onion (.5 of 1)
- Green pepper (1)
- Water (1 tbsp.)
- Cream (1 tbsp.)
- Black pepper (1 tsp.)
- Butter (3 tbsp.)

Preparation Technique:
1. Set the Air Fryer to 380° Fahrenheit. Chop the cauliflower and add to a blender to make rice. Dice the chicken fillet into bite-sized pieces.
2. Prepare the vegetables and combine each of the fixings.
3. Add the fryer basket and set the timer for 6-7 min.). Serve and enjoy.

Grilled Cheese Sandwiches

Yields Provided: 2 Servings
Ingredients:
- Sharp cheddar cheese (.5 cup)
- White bread or brioche (4 slices)
- Melted butter (.25 cup)

Preparation Technique:
1. Set the Air Fryer at 360° Fahrenheit.
2. Butter all slices of bread (both sides). Assemble each sandwich and arrange them in the fryer basket.
3. Prepare for 5-7 minutes and serve immediately for the best taste results.

Pita Bread - Pepperoni Sausage & Onion Pizza

Yields Provided: 1 Serving
Ingredients:
- Pizza sauce (1 tbsp.)
- Pita bread (1)
- Mozzarella cheese (.25 cup)
- Olive oil (1 spritz)
- Stainless-steel short-legged trivet (1)

Ingredients - The Toppings:
- Pepperoni (7 slices)
- Fresh minced garlic (.5 tsp.)
- Sausage (.25 cup)
- Thinly sliced onions (1 tbsp.)

Preparation Steps:
1. Heat the Air Fryer in advance to 350° Fahrenheit.
2. Spoon the sauce onto the bread.
3. Mince the garlic and thinly slice the onions. Toss on the toppings using a drizzle of oil.
4. Arrange it in the Air Fryer and place the trivet.
5. Set the timer for six minutes. Serve when it's nicely browned.

Roasted Veggie Pasta Salad

Yields Provided: 6 Servings
Ingredients:
- Yellow squash (1)
- Brown mushrooms (4 oz.)
- Zucchini (1)
- Red - Green - Orange bell peppers (1 each)
- Red onion (1)
- Fresh ground pepper and salt (1 pinch each)
- Italian seasoning (1 tsp.)
- Grape tomatoes (1 cup)
- Pitted Kalamata olives (.5 cup)
- Cooked Rigatoni or Penne Rigate (1 lb.)
- Olive oil (.25 cup)
- Fresh chopped basil (2 tbsp.)
- Balsamic vinegar (3 tbsp.)

Preparation Technique:
1. Preheat the Air Fryer to 380° Fahrenheit.
2. Cut the peppers into large chunks and slice the red onion. Slice the tomatoes and olives into halves. Cut the squash and zucchini into half-moons.
3. Put the mushrooms, peppers, red onion, squash, and zucchini in a large container. Drizzle with some of the oil, tossing well using the pepper, salt, and Italian seasoning.
4. Prepare in the Air Fryer until the veggies are softened - not mushy (12 to 15 min.). Toss the fixings in the basket about halfway through the cooking cycle for even frying.
5. Toss the cooked pasta, roasted veggies, olives, and tomatoes into a large container. Pour in the vinegar, and toss.
6. Keep it refrigerated until ready to serve — adding the fresh basil as serving time.

Stuffed Mushrooms

Yields Provided: 3 Servings
Ingredients:
- Portobello mushrooms (3)
- Minced garlic (1 tsp.)
- Medium diced onion (1)
- Grated mozzarella cheese (3 tbsp.)
- Chopped ham (2 slices)
- Diced tomato (1)
- Diced green pepper (1)
- Sea salt (.5 tsp.)
- Pepper (.25 tsp.)
- Olive oil (1 tbsp.)

Preparation Technique:
1. Set the Air Fryer temperature setting to 320° Fahrenheit.
2. Rinse, dry, and discard the stems from the portobello mushrooms. Drizzle with oil. Set aside for now.
3. Combine the cheese, tomato, onion, pepper, salt, garlic, bell peppers, and ham; stuff into the mushroom caps.
4. Arrange the mushrooms in the Air Fryer for 8 minutes.
5. Serve with your favorite main dish.

Twice Baked Loaded Air-Fried Potatoes

Yields Provided: 2 Servings
Ingredients:
- Olive oil (1 tsp.)
- Potato (14-16 oz.)
- Bacon bits (3 slices)
- Finely chopped green onion (1 tbsp. + .25 cup)
- Unsalted butter (1 tbsp.)
- Black pepper (.125 tsp.)
- Salt (.25 tsp.)
- Heavy cream (2 tbsp.)

Preparation Technique:
1. Cook the bacon about ten minutes - reserving the fat - and chop into ½-inch pieces.
2. Finely chop the onions.
3. Coat the potato with the oil and add it to the Air Fryer basket. Set the temperature to 400° Fahrenheit for 30 minutes. Turn the potato (spritzing with oil if needed), and cook for another 30 minutes. Cool for a minimum of 20 minutes.
4. When cooled, slice the potato lengthways. Scoop out the pulp leaving about ¼-inch borders to support the filling.
5. Whisk the scooped potato, bacon fat, bacon bits, .25 of a cup of the cheese, 1.5 tsp. of onions, pepper, salt, butter, and lastly the cream. Combine well.
6. Scoop the mixture into the prepared skins. Garnish with the cheese and place them in the Air Fryer.
7. Set the timer for 20 minutes or until the tops are browned.
8. Sprinkle the rest of the onions on top of the potato and serve.

Chapter 4: Poultry Choices

Breaded Chicken Tenderloin

Yields Provided: 4 Servings
Ingredients:
- Breadcrumbs (3.33 tbsp.)
- Butter/vegetable oil (2 tbsp.)
- Chicken tenderloins (8)
- Egg (1)

Preparation Technique:
1. Set the Air Fryer temperature to 356° Fahrenheit.
2. Combine the breadcrumbs and oil - stirring until the mixture crumbles.
3. Whisk the egg and run the chicken through the egg, shaking off the excess.
4. Dip each piece of the egged chicken into the crumbs to evenly coat.
5. Set the timer for 12 minutes. The time may vary according to the thickness of the chicken.

Buffalo Chicken Wings

Yields Provided: 2-3 Servings
Ingredients:
- Chicken wings (5 - approx. 14 oz.)
- Salt & black pepper (as desired)
- Cayenne pepper (2 tsp. or to taste)
- Red hot sauce (2 tbsp.)
- Melted butter (1 tbsp.)
- _Optional_: Garlic powder (.5 tsp.)

Preparation Technique:
1. Heat the Air Fryer temperature to reach 356° Fahrenheit.
2. Slice the wings into three sections (end tip, middle joint, and drumstick). Pat each one thoroughly dry using a paper towel.
3. Combine the pepper, salt, garlic powder, and cayenne pepper on a platter. Lightly cover the wings with the powder.
4. Arrange the chicken onto the wire rack and bake for 15 minutes, turning once at 7 minutes.
5. Combine the hot sauce, and melted butter in a dish to garnish the baked chicken when it is time to be served.

Chicken Curry

Yields Provided: 4 Servings

Ingredients:

- Chicken breast (1 lb.)
- Olive oil (1 tsp.)
- Onion (1)
- Garlic (2 tsp.)
- Lemongrass (1 tbsp.)
- Chicken stock (.5 cup)
- Apple cider vinegar (1 tbsp.)
- Coconut milk (.5 cup)
- Curry paste (2 tbsp.)

Preparation Technique:

1. Preheat the fryer to 365° Fahrenheit.
2. Dice the chicken into cubes. Peel and dice the onion and combine in the Air Fryer basket. Cook 5 minutes.
3. Remove and add the remainder of the fixings. Mix well and air-fry for another 10 minutes.
4. Serve for lunch or a quick and easy meal.

Chicken Hash

Yields Provided: 3 Servings
Ingredients:
- Chicken fillet (7 oz.)
- Cauliflower (6 oz.)
- Yellow onion (.5 of 1)
- Green pepper (1)
- Water (1 tbsp.)
- Cream (1 tbsp.)
- Black pepper (1 tsp.)
- Butter (3 tbsp.)

Preparation Technique:
1. Set the Air Fryer temperature to 380° Fahrenheit.
2. Chop the cauliflower and add to a blender to make rice. Slice the chicken into bite-sized pieces. Prepare the veggies and combine the fixings.
3. Add the fryer basket and cook until done (6-7 min.). Check it often to prevent scorching.
4. Serve and enjoy.

Chicken Parmesan

Yields Provided: 4 Servings

Ingredients:
- Chicken breast (2 - about 8 oz. each)
- Seasoned breadcrumbs (6 tbsp.)
- Grated parmesan cheese (2 tbsp.)
- Olive oil/melted butter (1 tbsp.)
- Reduced-fat mozzarella cheese (6 tbsp.)
- Marinara sauce (.5 cup)

Preparation Technique:
1. Set the Air Fryer at 360° Fahrenheit for 3 minutes.
2. Slice the chicken breasts into halves and into four thinner cutlets.
3. Combine the parmesan cheese and breadcrumbs in a bowl.
4. Melt the butter in another dish.
5. Lightly brush the butter onto the chicken, then dip into the breadcrumb mixture.
6. When the Air Fryer is ready, arrange two pieces in the basket and spray the top with a bit of cooking oil.
7. Fry for 6 minutes; turn and top each with 1 tbsp. sauce and 1.5 tbsp. of shredded mozzarella cheese.
8. Cook until the cheese is melted (3 min.).
9. Set aside and keep warm, repeat with the remaining two pieces.

Chicken Pot Pie

Yields Provided: 4 Servings

Ingredients:
- Chicken tenders (6)
- Potatoes (2)
- Condensed cream of celery soup (1.5 cups)
- Heavy cream (.75 cup)
- Thyme (1 sprig)
- Dried bay leaf (1 whole)
- Refrigerated buttermilk biscuits (5)
- Milk (1 tbsp.)
- Egg yolk (1)

Preparation Technique
1. Preheat the Air Fryer at 320° Fahrenheit.
2. Peel and dice the potatoes. Combine all of the fixings in a skillet except for the milk, egg yolk, and biscuits. Bring it to a boil using the medium-heat temperature setting.
3. Empty the mixture into the baking tin. Cover with a sheet of aluminum foil. Prepare a sling using a length of foil to make a handle. Place the pan into the fry basket using the sling. Cook for 15 minutes.
4. After the pie completes the cycle, prepare an egg wash using the milk and egg yolk.
5. Arrange the biscuits onto the baking pan and brush using the egg wash mixture. Set the timer for an additional ten minutes (300° Fahrenheit).
6. Serve when the biscuits are golden brown.

Chicken Strips

Yields Provided: 4 Servings
Ingredients:
- Chicken fillets (1 lb.)
- Paprika (1 tsp.)
- Heavy cream (1 tbsp.)
- Salt & pepper (.5 tsp.)
- Butter (as needed)

Preparation Technique:
1. Set the Air Fryer at 365° Fahrenheit.
2. Slice the fillets into strips and sprinkle using the salt and pepper.
3. Add a covering of butter to the basket.
4. Arrange the strips in the basket and air fry for 6 minutes.
5. Flip the strips and continue frying for another 5 minutes.
6. When done, sprinkle with the cream and paprika. Serve warm.

Chinese Wings

Yields Provided: 2 Servings
Ingredients:
- Chicken wings (4)
- Salt and pepper (as desired)
- Chinese spice (1 tbsp.)
- Mixed spices (1 tbsp.)
- Soy sauce (1 tbsp.)

Preparation Technique:
1. Warm up the fryer to 356° Fahrenheit.
2. Toss the seasonings into a large mixing bowl, whisking thoroughly. Sprinkle them over the wings until each piece is covered.
3. Put a layer of aluminum foil on the base of the Air Fryer (similar to how you cover a baking tray).
4. Add the chicken - sprinkling any remnants over the chicken. Cook for 15 minutes. Reduce the temperature setting to 392° Fahrenheit.
5. Flip the chicken over and cook another 15 minutes before serving with your favorite side dish.

Country-Style Chicken Tenders

Yields Provided: 3-4 Servings
Ingredients:
- Chicken tenders (.75 lb.)
- Olive oil (2 tbsp.)
- Salt (.5 tsp.)
- Beaten eggs (2)
- All-purpose flour (.5 cup)
- Seasoned breadcrumbs (.5 cup)
- Black pepper (1 tsp.)

Preparation Technique:
1. Preheat the Air Fryer temperature to reach 330° Fahrenheit.
2. Set up three separate dishes for the flour, eggs, and breadcrumbs.
3. Blend the oil, salt, pepper, and breadcrumbs. Mix well.
4. Toss the chicken tenders into the flour and the eggs. Coat evenly with the breadcrumbs. Shake the excess off before placing it in the Air Fryer basket.
5. Cook for 10 minutes at 330° Fahrenheit and increase to 390° Fahrenheit until they're a nicely browned (5 min.).

Fried Chicken Thighs

Yields Provided: 2 Servings
Ingredients:
- Chicken thighs - no skin (2)
- Fresh parsley (3 sprigs)
- Garlic powder – for dusting
- Salt & black pepper (as desired)
- Lemon (half if 1)
- Chili flakes (to taste)
- Fresh rosemary (1-2 sprigs)

Preparation Technique:
1. Rinse the thighs and drain between two paper towels.
2. Clean the rosemary sprigs and remove the stems. Chop or mince the parsley.
3. *Prepare the Marinade*: Combine the parsley, chili flakes, salt, pepper, garlic powder, rosemary leaves, and lemon juice. Add the thighs and marinate overnight in the fridge.
4. *Preheat the Air Fryer*: Set the fryer to 356° Fahrenheit. Grill for 12 minutes.

Herbal Chicken Wings

Yields Provided: 6 Servings
Ingredients:

- Chicken wings (4 lb.)
- Chopped thyme (1 tsp.)
- Minced garlic (6 cloves)
- Habanero (1 chopped)
- Fresh lime (1 juiced)
- Minced ginger (.5 tbsp.)
- Olive oil (1 tbsp.)
- Vinegar (2 tbsp. + .33 cup)
- Soy sauce (2 tbsp.)
- Brown sugar (1 tbsp.)
- Salt & White pepper (.5 tsp. each)
- Cinnamon (.25 tsp.)

Preparation Technique:

1. Program the Air Fryer to 390° Fahrenheit.
2. Mix each of the fixings in a bowl with a lid. Marinate for two hours.
3. Transfer the wings to the fryer basket (15 min.).
4. Serve any time.

Hot Chicken Wings

Yields Provided: 6-8 Servings
Ingredients:
- Chicken wings (2 lb.)
- Melted butter (3 tbsp.)
- Hot sauce (.25 cup)
- Salt

Ingredients - The Sauce:
- Hot sauce (4 tbsp.)
- Melted butter (3 tbsp.)

Preparation Technique:
1. Combine the melted butter, wings, hot sauce, and salt. Coat them well and pop into the refrigerator for two hours to marinate.
2. Set the oven temperature to 400° Fahrenheit.
3. Arrange the wings in the fryer basket and set the timer to fry for 12 minutes.
4. Combine the melted butter and hot sauce.
5. Transfer the wings from the basket and add to the hot sauce. Toss well.
6. Serve piping hot.

Jamaican Chicken Meatballs

Yields Provided: 10 Servings
Ingredients:
- Large chicken breasts (2)
- Onion (1 large)
- Chili powder (1 tsp.)
- Honey (2 tbsp.)
- Pepper and salt (as desired)
- Soy sauce (3 tbsp.)
- Thyme (1 tbsp.)
- Basil (1 tbsp.)
- Dry mustard (1 tbsp.)
- Cumin (1 tbsp.)
- Jerk paste (2 tsp.)

Preparation Technique:
1. Set the Air Fryer at 356° Fahrenheit.
2. Mince the chicken and onion. Using a blender, toss in the Jamaican seasonings and blend with the onions and chicken.
3. Prepare ten medium balls. Arrange the balls on a baking mat in the fryer.
4. When it's done, push them on a stick. Pour a portion of the sauce over the top of the prepared meatballs. Spice it up with the herbs of choice. Serve.
5. *Note*: Jerk paste is a combination of brown spices, peppers, ginger, and thyme.

Lemon & Rosemary Chicken

Yields Provided: 4-6 Servings
Ingredients:

- Chicken (1 lb.)

For the Marinade:

- Soy sauce (1 tbsp.)
- Olive oil (.5 tbsp.)
- Minced ginger (1 tsp.)

For the Sauce:

- Brown sugar (3 tbsp.)
- Lemon in skins (half of 1 - wedge-cut)
- Oyster sauce (1 tbsp.)

Optional: Fresh rosemary (0.5 oz.)

Preparation Technique:

1. Leave the skin on the rosemary and chop.
2. Blend all of the marinade fixings.Pour over the chicken. Store it all in the fridge for about 30 minutes.
3. Pour the marinade and chicken in a baking container and set the timer for six minutes in the Air Fryer at 392° Fahrenheit.
4. Blend all of the sauce components (minus the lemon). Pour the mixture over the chicken when it is about half-baked.
5. Place the lemon wedges in the pan evenly and squeeze so the zest will heighten the flavor of the chicken.
6. Continue baking for 13 minutes turning to ensure all of the pieces are browned evenly.

Old Bay Chicken Wings

Yields Provided: 4 Servings
Ingredients
- Chicken wing parts (3 lb.)
- Old Bay Seasoning (1 tbsp.)
- Potato starch (.75 cup)
- Butter (.5 cup)
- Fresh lemons
- True Lemon (1 tsp.) or more juice of a lemon (as desired)

Preparation Technique:
1. Heat the Air Fryer in advance to reach 360° Fahrenheit.
2. Rinse and dry the wings with several paper towels.
3. Whisk the seasoning and potato starch. Add the wings and toss to coat. Set the timer for 35 minutes. Shake the basket often.
4. Melt the butter and add it along with the True Lemon. Add it to the hot wings.
5. Stir and add the rest of the lemon butter and lemons for squeezing.

Orange Wings

Yields Provided: 2 Servings

Ingredients:

- Orange (1 - zest & juiced)
- Chicken wings (6)
- Worcestershire sauce (1.5 tbsp.)
- Sugar (1 tbsp.)
- Herbs: Sage, thyme, parsley, oregano, basil, mint, etc.
- Pepper (as desired)

Preparation Technique:

1. Prepare the wings and pour the orange juice and zest into a bowl. Mix in the rest of the fixings and rub it in well. Marinate for 30 minutes.
2. Set the temperature on the Air Fryer to 356° Fahrenheit.
3. Combine the wings and juices together. Add to the fryer basket for 20 minutes.
4. Remove the wings from the fryer and discard the zest and brush half of the sauce over the wings. Return to the fryer and cook an additional ten minutes.
5. Add the wings to a serving platter and serve.

Rotisserie-Style - Whole Chicken

Yields Provided: 4 Servings
Ingredients:

- Olive oil (as needed)
- Whole chicken (6-7 lb.)
- Seasoned salt

Preparation Technique:

1. Clean and dry the chicken and coat with the oil. Season with the salt.
2. Arrange the chicken in the Air Fryer – skin-side down.
3. Cook at 350° Fahrenheit for 30 minutes. Flip it over and continue cooking another 30 minutes.
4. Serve when it's to your liking.

Tarragon Chicken

Yields Provided: 1 Serving
Ingredients:

- Skinless & boneless chicken breast (1)
- Kosher salt (.125 tsp.)
- Freshly cracked black pepper (.125 tsp.)
- Unsalted butter (.5 tsp.)
- Dried tarragon (.25 tsp.)

Preparation Technique:

1. Set the temperature in advance to reach 390° Fahrenheit.
2. Place the chicken in aluminum foil (12x14). Add the tarragon and butter with a sprinkle of salt and pepper.
3. Loosely wrap the foil for minimal airflow. Air fry for 12 minutes in the basket. Serve.

Turkey Options

Avocado & Turkey Burrito

Yields Provided: 2 Servings
Ingredients:
- Eggs (4)
- Salt & black pepper (as desired)
- Tortillas (2)
- Salsa (4 tbsp.)
- Cooked turkey breast (8 slices)
- Sliced avocado (.5 cup)
- Mozzarella cheese (.25 cup - grated)
- Sliced red bell pepper (.5 of 1)

Preparation Technique:
1. Set the temperataure setting at 390° Fahrenheit.
2. Spritz the Air Fryer tray with a portion of cooking oil spray. Whisk the eggs with the pepper and salt and add to the fryer basket.
3. Prepare for five minutes. Scrape the bowl and add the eggs onto the tortillas.
4. Layer the turkey, avocado, peppers, cheese, and salsa. Roll it up slowly.
5. Spray the Air Fryer and arrange the burritos in the basket. Set the timer for 5 minutes.
6. Serve warm.

Mustard-Glazed Turkey Breast

Yields Provided: 6 Servings
Ingredients:
- Olive oil (2 tsp.)
- Whole turkey breast (5 lb.)
- Salt (1 tsp.)
- Dried thyme (1 tsp.)
- Butter (1 tsp.)
- Freshly cracked black pepper (.5 tsp.)
- Smoked paprika (.5 tsp.)
- Dried sage (.5 tsp.)
- Maple syrup (.25 tsp.)
- Dijon mustard (2 tbsp.)

Preparation Technique:
1. Warm the fryer to 350° Fahrenheit.
2. Prepare the turkey with a spritz of olive oil.
3. Mix the sage, salt, thyme, pepper, and paprika as a rub. Use it as a coating for the turkey.
4. Arrange the breast in the fryer basket and set the timer for 25 minutes. Rotate it on its side and fry another 12 minutes. It's done when it reaches 165° Fahrenheit – internal temperature.
5. In the meantime, whisk the butter, syrup, and mustard in a saucepan. Turn the breast again and brush using the glaze. Give it a final five minutes until crispy.
6. Cover using a foil tent for five minutes, slice, and serve.

Reuben Roasted Turkey

Yields Provided: 2 Servings
Ingredients:
- Rye bread (4 slices)
- Skinless – roasted turkey breast (8 slices)
- Coleslaw (4 tbsp.)
- Swiss cheese (8 slices)
- Salted butter (2 tbsp.)
- Russian dressing (2 tbsp.)

Preparation Technique:
1. Prepare two slices of the bread on one side with butter and place them – butter side down - on the cutting board.
2. In layers, arrange the turkey, cheese, coleslaw, and Russian dressing on top of the two slices of bread. Fold them together to make one sandwich.
3. Add the sandwich to the Air Fryer basket.
4. Choose the bake icon setting (310° Fahrenheit for 12 min.).
5. After six minutes, flip the sandwich, and continue until browned.
6. When done, slice and serve.

Roast Turkey Breast

Yields Provided: 8-10 Servings

Ingredients:
- Olive oil (2 tbsp.)
- Freshly cracked black pepper (1 tbsp.)
- Bone-in turkey breast (8 lb.)
- Sea salt (2 tbsp.)

Preparation Technique:
1. Warm the Air Fryer to 360° Fahrenheit.
2. Rub the turkey with oil and the seasonings.
3. Put the turkey in the fryer basket for 20 minutes.
4. When done, flip it over and adjust the cooking time for another 20 minutes (also at 360° Fahrenheit).
5. The breast of turkey is done when it indicates 165° Fahrenheit when tested using a meat thermometer.
6. Wait for a minimum of 20 minutes before serving.

Chapter 5: Pork & Lamb Specialties

Pork Options

<u>Bacon-Wrapped Pork Tenderloin</u>

Yields Provided: 4-6 Servings
Ingredients:
- Bacon (3-4 strips)
- Pork tenderloin (1 lb.)
- Dijon mustard (1-2 tbsp.)

Preparation Technique:
1. Coat the tenderloin with the mustard and wrap with the bacon.
2. Set the Air Fryer temperature at 360° Fahrenheit for 15 minutes. Flip and cook 10-15 more minutes.
3. Serve with your favorite sides.

Balsamic Smoked Raspberry Pork Chops

Yields Provided: 4 Servings

Ingredients:

- Large eggs (2)
- Finely chopped pecans (1 cup)
- Japanese – panko breadcrumbs (1 cup)
- 2% milk (.25 cup)
- All-purpose flour (.25 cup)
- Smoked bone-in pork chops (4)
- Balsamic vinegar (.33 cup)
- Seedless raspberry jam (2 tbsp.)
- Brown sugar (2 tbsp.)
- Frozen orange juice concentrate - thawed (1 tbsp.)

Preparation Technique:

1. Set the Air Fryer at 400° Fahrenheit. Spritz the basket with cooking oil spray.
2. Whisk the milk and eggs in one dish and combine the pecans and breadcrumbs in another.
3. Prepare in batches. Dip in the flour, shaking off the excess. Dip them into the egg mix.
4. Prepare in single layers in the fryer 12-15 minutes, turning about halfway through the cooking cycle.
5. Combine the rest of the fixings in a saucepan, bringing it to a boil. Simmer 6 to 8 minutes until thickened. Serve over the chops.

Crispy Breaded Pork Chops

Yields Provided: 6 Servings
Ingredients:
- Center-cut boneless chops (6 - 3/4-inch each)
- Large egg (1)
- Kosher salt (.75 tsp.)
- Panko crumbs (.5 cup)
- Crushed cornflakes (.33 cup)
- Sweet paprika (1.25 tsp.)
- Grated parmesan cheese (2 tbsp.)
- Onion (.5 tsp.)
- Garlic (.5 tsp.)
- Chili powder (.25 tsp.)
- Freshly cracked black pepper (.125 tsp.)

Preparation Technique:
1. Set the Air Fryer to reach 400° Fahrenheit. Lightly spray the basket with cooking spray.
2. Shake the salt over the chops.
3. Mix the cornflake crumbs, panko, salt, pepper, and chili powder.
4. Whisk the egg in another container and dip the pork. Next, dip in the crumb mixture and add to the basket.
5. Prepare in two batches. Cook for 12 minutes – flipping halfway through the cycle. Spritz both sides of the chops before browning.

Roast Pork Loin with Red Potatoes

Yields Provided: 2 Servings
Ingredients:
- Large red potatoes (2)
- Pork loin (2 lb.)
- Pepper (1 tsp.)
- Salt (1 tsp.)
- Parsley (1 tsp.)
- Red pepper flakes (.5 tsp.)
- Garlic powder (.5 tsp.)
- A balsamic glaze from cooking

Preparation Technique:
1. Dice the potatoes.
2. Combine all of the seasonings and sprinkle over the potatoes and pork.
3. Arrange the pork and then the potatoes in the Air Fryer.
4. Secure the top and choose the roast button. Set the timer for 25 minutes.
5. When done, wait for a few minutes before slicing.
6. In the meanwhile, pour the roasted potatoes into the serving dishes.
7. Slice the pork loin into 4 to 5 sections.
8. Use a balsamic glaze over the pork and serve.

Southern Fried Chops

Yields Provided: 5 Servings
Ingredients:
- Pork chops (4)
- Buttermilk (3 tbsp.)
- All-purpose flour (.25 cup)
- Seasoning salt & black pepper (as desired)

Preparation Technique:
1. Rinse and dry the chops using a paper towel. Season using the pepper and seasoning salt.
2. Drizzle the chops with the buttermilk and toss into a zipper-type bag with the flour. Marinate for 30 minutes.
3. Arrange the chops in the fryer (stacking is okay). Spritz using a cooking oil spray.
4. Air fry for 15 minutes (380° Fahrenheit). Flip after the first 10 minutes.
5. Serve with your favorite side dishes.

Stuffed Pork Chops

Yields Provided: 3 Servings

Ingredients:
- Salt & Pepper (as desired)
- Thick-cut pork chops (3)
- Chopped mushrooms (7)
- Lemon juice (1 tbsp.)
- Pepper & salt (as desired)
- Almond flour (1 tbsp.)

Preparation Technique:
1. Set the Air Fryer temperature to reach 350° Fahrenheit.
2. Season the meat using the pepper and salt.
3. Arrange the chops in the Air Fryer. Set the timer for 15 minutes.
4. In a skillet, sauté the mushrooms for three minutes using a spritz lemon juice.
5. Toss in the flour and herbs and sauté for about four minutes and set aside.
6. Cut five sheets of foil for the chops. Arrange the chops on the foil and add some of the mushroom fixings.
7. Fold the foil to seal the chop and juices. Place the chops in the Air Fryer for 30 minutes.
8. Serve with a side salad.

Lamb Options

Lamb Meatballs

Yields Provided: 4 Servings
Ingredients:
- Coriander (1 tbsp.)
- Mint (1 tbsp.)
- Ground lamb (1 lb.)
- Egg white (1)
- Turkey (4 oz.)
- Salt (.5 tsp.)
- Minced garlic cloves (2)
- Parsley (2 tbsp.)
- Olive oil (1 tbsp.)

Preparation Technique:
1. Warm the Air Fryer in advance to 320° Fahrenheit.
2. Chop the mint and coriander.
3. Mix all of the fixings and shape into small meatballs.
4. Arrange in the Air Fryer and set the timer for 15 minutes.
5. When ready, serve it with your favorite sauce.

Lamb Ribs - Saltimbocca

Yields Provided: 4 Servings

Ingredients:
- Mozzarella cheese (2 balls)
- Lamb racks (2 lb.)
- Thinly sliced pieces of prosciutto (4)
- Sage leaves (4)
- Olive oil (2 tbsp.)

Preparation Technique:
1. Heat the Air Fryer to reach 350° Fahrenheit.
2. Slice the racks of lamb into quarters. Slice a deep pocket in each of the chops. Stuff with thinly sliced cheese pieces.
3. Place a sage leaf on top and wrap with sliced prosciutto.
4. Spritz using one tablespoon of the oil. Set the timer for 15 minutes.
5. Transfer to a platter and serve.

Roasted Rack Of Lamb with A Macadamia Crust

Yields Provided: 4-5 Servings
Ingredients:
- Garlic (1 clove)
- Olive oil (1 tbsp.)
- Pepper and salt (as desired)
- Rack of lamb (1.75 lb.)

Ingredients - The Crust:
- Macadamia nuts (3 oz. unsalted)
- Fresh rosemary (1 tbsp.)
- Breadcrumbs (1 tbsp.)
- Egg (1)

Preparation Technique:
1. Warm the Air Fryer to 220° Fahrenheit.
2. Dice the garlic clove into tiny bits. Make the garlic oil by mixing the garlic and oil. Brush the lamb and flavor using salt and pepper.
3. Finely chop the nuts into a bowl. Blend in the rosemary and breadcrumbs. Beat/whisk the egg in another dish.
4. Dredge the lamb through the egg mixture and coat with the macadamia crust topping.
5. Arrange the rack of lamb in the Air Fryer basket—setting the timer for 30 minutes.
6. Lastly; raise the heat to 390° Fahrenheit and set the timer for an additional five minutes.
7. Take the lamb from the fryer and wait for about ten minutes. Cover with a tent of aluminum foil.
8. *Substitutes to Consider:* You can use hazelnuts, pistachios, cashews, or almonds.

Spicy Lamb Sirloin Steak

Yields Provided: 4 Servings
Ingredient List:
- Boneless lamb sirloin steaks (1 lb.)
- Onion (half of 1)
- Salt (1 tsp.)
- Ginger (4 slices)
- Garlic (5 cloves)
- Ground fennel (1 tsp.)
- Ground cardamom (.5 tsp.)
- Garam masala (1 tsp.)
- Cayenne (.5 - 1 tsp.)
- Cinnamon (1 tsp.)

Preparation Steps:
1. Toss in all of the fixings into a blender, except the lamb chops.
2. Mix until the onion is finely minced, and everything is blended (3-4 min.).
3. Arrange the lamb chops into a large container. Use a sharp knife to slash the meat and fat. Add the blended spice paste. Combine thoroughly.
4. Put the mixture in the fridge for a minimum of 30 minutes or up to 24 hours.
5. Warm the Air Fryer. Set the fryer to 330° Fahrenheit for 15 minutes and add the lamb steaks in the fryer basket. Cook, flipping halfway through.
6. Use a meat thermometer to test the meat to make sure it's reached an internal temperature of 150° Fahrenheit for medium-well. Serve.

Chapter 6: Seafood & Fish

Air-Fried Crab Sticks

Yields Provided: 2-3 Servings
Ingredients:
- Crab sticks (1 package)
- Cooking oil spray (as needed)

Preparation Technique:
1. Take each of the sticks out of the package and unroll until flat. Tear the sheets into thirds.
2. Arrange them on a plate and lightly spritz using cooking spray. Set the timer for 10 minutes.
3. *Note*: If you shred the crab meat; you can cut the time in half, but they will also easily fall through the holes in the basket.

Breaded Cod Sticks

Yields Provided: 5 Servings
Ingredients:
- Milk (3 tbsp.)
- Large eggs (2)
- Breadcrumbs (2 cups)
- Salt (.25 tsp.)
- Black pepper (.5 tsp.)
- Almond flour (1 cup)
- Cod (1 lb.)

Preparation Technique:
1. Set the Air Fryer at 350° Fahrenheit.
2. Prepare three bowls; 1 with the milk and eggs; 1 with the pepper, salt, and breadcrumbs; and another with almond flour.
3. Dip the sticks in the flour, egg mixture, and lastly - the breadcrumbs.
4. Arrange in the basket and set the timer for 12 minutes – shaking halfway through the cooking process.
5. Serve with your favorite sauce.

Breaded Fried Shrimp

Yields Provided: 4 Servings
Ingredients:
- Raw shrimp (1 lb.)
- Egg white (3 tbsp. or 1 egg)
- All-purpose flour (.5 cup)
- Panko breadcrumbs (.75 cup)
- Paprika (1 tsp.)
- Pepper & salt (as desired)
- McCormick's Grill Mates Montreal Chicken Seasoning
- Cooking oil spray (as needed)

Ingredients - The Sauce:
- Sriracha (2 tbsp.)
- Plain non-fat Greek yogurt (.33 cup)
- Sweet chili sauce (.25 cup)

Preparation Technique:
1. Peel and devein the shrimp.
2. Set the temperature of the Air Fryer to 400° Fahrenheit.
3. Add the seasonings to the shrimp.
4. Use three bowls for the breadcrumbs, egg whites, and flour.
5. Dip the shrimp into the flour, the egg, and the breadcrumbs.
6. Lightly spritz the shrimp with the cooking spray and add to the fryer basket for four minutes.
7. Flip the shrimp and continue cooking for another four minutes.
8. Combine all of the fixings for the sauce and toss with the shrimp before serving.

Cajun Salmon

Yields Provided: 1-2 Servings

Ingredients:
- Salmon fillet – ¾-inch thick (1)
- Juice of ¼ lemon
- *For Breading*: Cajun seasoning for coating
- *Optional*: Sprinkle of sugar

Preparation Technique:
1. Warm the Air Fryer to 356° Fahrenheit (approx. 5 min.).
2. Rinse and pat the salmon dry. Thoroughly coat the fish with the coating mix.
3. Arrange the fillet in the fryer basket and set the timer for seven minutes with the skin side facing upward.
4. Serve with a drizzle of lemon.

Cajun Shrimp

Yields Provided: 4-6 Servings
Ingredients:
- Olive oil (1 tbsp.)
- Old Bay seasoning (.5 tsp.)
- Tiger shrimp (1.25 lb. or 16-20)
- Smoked paprika (.25 tsp.)
- Cayenne pepper (.25 tsp.)
- Salt (1 pinch)

Preparation Technique:
1. Heat the Air Fryer to reach 390° Fahrenheit.
2. Coat the shrimp using the oil and spices.
3. Place the shrimp in the fryer basket and set the timer for five minutes.
4. Serve with your favorite side dish.

Coconut Shrimp

Yields Provided: 3 Servings

Ingredients:
- Coconut – unsweetened & dried (1 cup)
- Gluten-free breadcrumbs (1 cup)
- Shrimp (12 large)
- Gluten-free flour (1 cup)
- Egg white (1 cup)
- Cornstarch (1 tbsp.)

Preparation Technique:
1. Set the Air Fryer to 350° Fahrenheit.
2. Select a shallow platter and combine coconut and the breadcrumbs.
3. In another bowl, mix the flour and cornstarch. Break the egg into a small bowl.
4. Coat the shrimp with the egg white, flour, and lastly the breadcrumbs.
5. Place in the fryer basket and fry for 10 minutes.
6. Serve with your favorite sides or as a quick snack.

Creamy Salmon

Yields Provided: 2 Servings
Ingredients:

- Salmon (.75 lb. - 6 pieces)
- Salt (1 pinch)
- Olive oil (1 tbsp.)
- Chopped dill (1 tbsp.)
- Sour cream (3 tbsp.)
- Plain yogurt (1.75 oz.)

Preparation Technique:

1. Program the temperature setting on the Air Fryer to 285° Fahrenheit.
2. Pour oil into the fryer basket. Shake the salt over the salmon and add it to the fryer basket. Air fry for 10 minutes.
3. Whisk the yogurt, dill, and salt.
4. Serve the salmon with the sauce and your favorite sides.

Crispy Halibut

Yields Provided: 4 Servings
Ingredients:
- Halibut fillets (4)
- Fresh chives (.25 cup)
- Fresh parsley (.5 cup)
- Fresh dill (.25 cup)
- Black pepper & sea salt (to your liking)
- Pork rinds (.75 cup)
- Extra-virgin olive oil (1 tbsp.)
- Finely grated lemon zest (1 tbsp.)

Preparation Technique:
1. Warm the Air Fryer to reach 390° Fahrenheit.
2. Chop the chives, dill, and parsley. Combine all of the dry fixings – parsley, pork rinds, chives, dill, lemon zest, black pepper, sea salt, and olive oil.
3. Rinse the halibut well and let them drain well on paper towels.
4. Prepare a baking tin to fit in the cooker. Spoon the rinds over the fish and press in.
5. Add the prepared fillets in the fryer for 30 minutes.

Dill Salmon

Yields Provided: 4 Servings
Ingredients:
- Salmon (4 - 6-oz. pieces or 1.5 lb.)
- Salt (1 pinch)
- Olive oil (2 tsp.)

Ingredients - The Sauce:
- Sour cream (.5 cup)
- Non-fat Greek yogurt (.5 cup)
- Dill (2 finely chopped tbsp.)
- Salt (1 pinch)

Preparation Technique:
1. Preheat the Air Fryer prior to baking time (270° Fahrenheit).
2. Chop the salmon into the four portions. Drizzle with about half of the oil (1 tsp.). Flavor with a pinch of salt and add to the basket for about 20-23 minutes.
3. Lastly, blend the yogurt, salt, sour cream, and dill in a mixing container. Pour the sauce over the cooked salmon with a pinch of chopped dill.

E-Z Catfish

Yields Provided: 3 Servings
Ingredients:
- Olive oil (1 tbsp.)
- Seasoned fish fry (.25 cup)
- Catfish fillets (4)

Preparation Technique:
1. Prepare the fryer to 400° Fahrenheit.
2. First, rinse the fish, and pat dry with a paper towel.
3. Dump the seasoning into a large zip-type baggie. Add the fish and shake to cover each fillet. Spray with a spritz of cooking oil spray. Add to the basket.
4. Set the timer for ten minutes. Flip, and reset the timer for ten more minutes. Flip once more and cook for two to three minutes.
5. Once it reaches the desired crispiness, transfer to a plate to serve.

Fish & Chips

Yields Provided: 4 Servings
Ingredients:

- Catfish fillets or similar fish (2)
- Wholemeal bread for breadcrumbs (3 slices)
- Medium beaten egg (1)
- Bag tortilla chips (0.88 oz. or approximately/25g)
- Juice and rind of 1 lemon
- Pepper and salt
- Parsley (1 tbsp.)

Preparation Technique:

1. Warm the fryer before baking time to reach 356° Fahrenheit.
2. Zest and juice the lemon.
3. Slice the fillets into four pieces ready for cooking. Season each one with the lemon juice and set aside for a few minutes.
4. Use a food processor to mix the tortillas, parsley, pepper, breadcrumbs, and lemon zest.
5. Whisk the egg and egg wash the fish. Run it through the crumb mixture. Place them onto the baking tray and cook until crispy.
6. Preparation time is ten minutes with a total cooking time of fifteen minutes; so, wait patiently to enjoy.

Fish Nuggets

Yields Provided: 4 Servings
Ingredients:
- Cod fillet (1 lb.)
- Eggs (3)
- Olive oil (4 tbsp.)
- Almond flour (1 cup)
- Gluten-free breadcrumbs (1 cup)
- Salt (1 tsp.)

Preparation Technique:
1. Set the temperature of the Air Fryer at 390° Fahrenheit.
2. Cut the cod into nuggets.
3. Prepare three dishes. Beat the eggs in one. Combine the salt, oil, and breadcrumbs in another. The last one will be almond flour.
4. Cover each of the nuggets using the flour, a dip in the eggs, and the breadcrumbs.
5. Arrange the prepared nuggets in the basket and set the timer for 20 minutes. Serve.

Fish Tacos

Yields Provided: 6 Servings
Ingredients:
- Tempura batter (1 cup) made from:
    - Flour (1 cup)
    - Cornstarch (1 tbsp.)
    - Salt & pepper (1 pinch each)
- Cold seltzer water (.5 cup)
- Salsa (.5 cup)
- Coleslaw (1 cup)
- White pepper (1 tsp.)
- Chopped cilantro (2 tbsp.)
- Guacamole (.5 cup)
- Lemon wedges (1)

Preparation Technique:
1. Prep the tempura batter using the salt, pepper. cornstarch, and flour.
2. Slice the cod into two-ounce pieces (6 pieces) and sprinkle using the salt and pepper.
3. Use the batter) to coat the cod. Dredge them in the panko.
4. Use the French fry setting and set the timer for ten minutes. Turn after five minutes.
5. Top each portion with coleslaw, salsa, guacamole, cilantro, or lemon juice.

Ginger Cod Steaks

Yields Provided: 2 Servings
Ingredients:
- Large cod steaks (2 slices)
- Turmeric powder (.25 tsp.)
- Ginger powder (.5 tsp.)
- Garlic powder (.5 tsp.)
- Salt & pepper (1 pinch)
- Plum sauce (1 tbsp.)
- Ginger slices (as desired)
- Kentucky Kernel Seasoned Flour (+) Corn flour (1 part of each)

Preparation Technique:
1. Dry off the steaks and marinate using the pepper, salt, ginger powder, and turmeric powder for a few minutes.
2. Lightly coat the steaks with the corn flour/Kentucky mix.
3. Set the temperature in the fryer to 356° Fahrenheit for 15 minutes and increase to 400° Fahrenheit for 5 minutes. (Time may vary depending on the size of the cod.)
4. Prepare the sauce in a wok. Brown the ginger slices and remove from the heat. Stir in the plum sauce adding water to thin as needed.
5. Serve the steaks with a drizzle of the prepared sauce.

Grilled Shrimp

Yields Provided: 4 Servings
Ingredients:

- Medium shrimp/prawns (8)
- Melted butter (1 tbsp.)
- Rosemary (1 sprig)
- Pepper and salt (as desired)
- Minced garlic cloves (3)

Preparation Technique:

1. Combine all of the fixings in a mixing bowl. Toss well and arrange in the fryer basket.
2. Set the timer for 7 minutes (356° Fahrenheit) and serve.

Honey & Sriracha Tossed Calamari

Yields Provided: 1-2 Servings

Ingredients:
- Calamari tubes - tentacles if you prefer (.5 lb.)
- Club soda (1 cup)
- Four (1 cup)
- Salt - red pepper & black pepper (2 dashes each)
- Honey (.5 cup) + 1-2 tbsp. Sriracha
- Red pepper flakes (2 shakes)

Preparation Technique:
1. Fully rinse the calamari and blot it dry using a bunch of paper towels. Slice into rings (.25-inch wide). Toss the rings into a bowl. Pour in the club soda and stir until all are submerged. Wait for about 10 minutes.
2. Sift the salt, flour, red & black pepper. Set aside for now.
3. Dredge the calamari into the flour mixture and set on a platter until ready to fry.
4. Spritz the basket of the Air Fryer with a small amount of cooking oil spray. Arrange the calamari in the basket, careful not to crowd it too much.
5. Set the temperature at 375° Fahrenheit and the timer for 11 minutes.
6. Shake the basket twice during the cooking process, loosening any rings that may stick.
7. Remove from the basket, toss with the sauce, and return to the fryer for two more minutes.
8. Serve with additional sauce as desired.
9. Make the sauce by combining honey, sriracha, and red pepper flakes in a small bowl, mix until fully combined.

Lemon Fish

Yields Provided: 4 Servings

Ingredients:
- Water (.5 cup + 3 tbsp.)
- Sugar (.25 cup)
- Juice of 1 lemon
- Green chili sauce (2 tsp.)
- Salt (to your liking)
- Egg white (1)
- Corn flour slurry (4 tsp.)
- Red chili sauce (1 tsp.)
- Lettuce (2-3 leaves)
- Catfish (2 - cut into 4 pieces)
- Oil (2 tsp.)

Preparation Technique:
1. Boil the water and sugar in a saucepan. Slice the lemon and place it in a dish.
2. Add the egg white, oil, chili sauce, salt, and flour in a bowl, mixing well. Add three tablespoons of water and whisk to make a smooth slurry batter.
3. Sprinkle flour onto a plate. Dip in the batter and then the flour.
4. Lightly grease the Air Fryer basket with a spritz of cooking oil spray and heat to reach 356° Fahrenheit.
5. Arrange the fillets in the basket and cook for 15 to 20 minutes until crispy.
6. Add salt to the pan and stir well. Add the corn flour slurry and mix it again. Blend in the red sauce juice, and lemon slices, mixing well and cooking until thickened.
7. Remove the fish from the basket, brush with a spritz of oil, and place back into the pan. Cook for about five additional minutes.
8. Tear the leaves apart to make a serving bed. Add the

fish and pour the lemon sauce over the top of the fish.
Serve.

Oregano Clams

Yields Provided: 4 Servings

Ingredients:
- Shucked clams (2 dozen)
- Dried oregano (1 tsp.)
- Chopped parsley (.25 cup)
- Grated parmesan cheese (.25 cup)
- Unseasoned breadcrumbs (1 cup)
- Melted butter (4 tbsp.)
- Minced garlic cloves (3)
- *For the Pan*: Sea salt (1 cup)

Preparation Technique:
1. Warm up the Air Fryer a few minutes at 400° Fahrenheit.
2. Mince the garlic and combine with the breadcrumbs, oregano, parsley, parmesan cheese, and melted butter in a medium mixing bowl.
3. Using a heaping tablespoon of the crumb mixture, add it to the clams.
4. Fill the insert with salt, arrange the clams inside, and air fry for three minutes.
5. Garnish with fresh parsley and lemon wedges.

Salmon Croquettes

Yields Provided: 4 Servings

Ingredients:
- Red salmon (1 lb. can)
- Breadcrumbs (1 cup)
- Vegetable oil (.33 cup)
- Chopped parsley (half of 1 bunch)
- Eggs (2)

Preparation Technique:
1. Set the Air Fryer at 392° Fahrenheit.
2. Drain and mash the salmon. Whisk and add the eggs and parsley.
3. In another dish, mix the breadcrumbs and oil.
4. Prepare 16 croquettes using the breadcrumb mixture.
5. Arrange in the preheated fryer basket for seven minutes.
6. Serve.

Salmon Patties

Yields Provided: 6-8 Servings
Ingredients:
- Salmon fillet (1 portion - approx. 7 oz.)
- Russet potatoes (3 large - approx. 14 oz.)
- Frozen veggies (.33 cup)
- Dill sprinkles (2 pinches)
- Salt and pepper (1 dash each)
- Egg (1)

Ingredients - The Coating:
- Breadcrumbs
- Olive oil spray

Preparation Steps:
1. Warm the Air Fryer to reach 356° Fahrenheit.
2. Peel and chop the potatoes into small bits. Boil for about ten minutes.
   Mash and place in the refrigerator to cool.
3. Grill the salmon for five minutes. Flake it apart and set it aside for now.
4. Combine all of the fixings and shape into patties. Evenly coat with the breadcrumbs, and spray with a bit of olive oil spray.
5. Place in the fryer for 10-12 minutes.

Shrimp Scampi

Yields Provided: 4 Servings

Ingredients:
- Butter (4 tbsp.)
- Minced garlic (1 tbsp.)
- Dried chives (1 tsp.) or Chopped chives (1 tbsp.)
- Red pepper flakes (2 tsp.)
- Dried (1 tsp.) or Minced basil leaves plus more for sprinkling (1 tbsp.)
- Lemon juice (1 tbsp.)
- Chicken stock or white wine (2 tbsp.)
- Defrosted shrimp (1 lb. or about 21-25 count)
- *Also Needed*: 6x3 metal pan & silicone mitts

Preparation Technique:
1. Set the Air Fryer at 330° Fahrenheit. Warm the pan at the same time.
2. Add the garlic, pepper flakes, and butter to the hot pan. Sauté for two minutes, stirring once to infuse the garlic.
3. Open the Air Fryer, stirring gently.
4. Set the timer for 5 minutes, stirring once.
5. At this point, the butter should be melted.
6. Remove the pan with oven mitts. The shrimp will continue cooking, but let it sit on the countertop to cool.
7. Stir well and dust with a layer of freshly chopped basil leaves.

Teriyaki Glazed Halibut Steak

Yields Provided: 3 Servings
Ingredients:
- Halibut steak (1 lb.)

Ingredients - The Marinade:
- Low-sodium soy sauce (.66 cup)
- Mirin Japanese cooking wine (.5 cup)
- Sugar (.25 cup)
- Orange juice (.25 cup)
- Lime juice (2 tbsp.)
- Ground ginger (.25 tsp.)
- Crushed red pepper flakes (.25 tsp.)
- Smashed garlic (1 clove)

Preparation Technique:
1. Warm the Air Fryer at 390° Fahrenheit.
2. Mix all of the marinade fixings in a saucepan, bringing it to a boil. Lower the heat setting to medium and cool.
3. Pour half of the marinade in a plastic bag with the halibut and zip it closed. Marinate in the refrigerator for about 30 minutes.
4. Air fry the halibut for 10-12 minutes. Brush using the remaining glaze over the steak.
5. Serve with a bed of rice. Add a little basil or mint or basil for extra flavoring.

Tomato & Basil Scallops

Yields Provided: 2 Servings
Ingredients:
- Jumbo sea scallops (8)
- Frozen spinach (12 oz.)
- Vegetable oil to spray (as needed)
- Tomato paste (1 tbsp.)
- Heavy whipping cream (.75 cup)
- Chopped fresh basil (1 tbsp.)
- Minced garlic (1 tsp.)
- Black pepper & salt (.5 tsp. each)
- Additional salt and pepper - to season scallops
- *Also Needed:* 7-inch heat-proof pan

Preparation Technique:
1. Thaw and drain the spinach.
2. Spray the pan. Scoop a layer of spinach in the pan.
3. Spray both sides of the scallops with vegetable oil. Dust with pepper and salt. Arrange the scallops in the pan on top of the spinach.
4. Combine the basil, garlic, cream, tomato paste, salt, and pepper. Pour the mixture over the spinach and scallops.
5. Set the Air Fryer at 350° Fahrenheit for 10 minutes until the scallops are cooked thoroughly. The sauce will also be bubbling.
6. Serve immediately.

Chapter 7: Beef Favorites

Beef & Potato Surprise

Yields Provided: 4 Servings
Ingredients:
- Mashed potatoes (3 cups)
- Ground beef (1 lb.)
- Eggs (2)
- Garlic powder (2 tbsp.)
- Sour cream (1 cup)
- Freshly cracked black pepper (as desired)
- Salt (1 pinch)

Preparation Technique:
1. Set the Air Fryer to reach 390° Fahrenheit.
2. Combine all of the fixings in a mixing container. Scoop it into a heat-safe dish.
3. Arrange in the fryer to cook for two minutes.
4. Serve for a special luncheon.

Beef Bulgogi Burgers

Yields Provided: 4 Servings
Ingredients - The Burgers:

- Gochujang (2 tbsp.)
- Ground beef (1 lb.)
- Minced garlic (2 tsp.)
- Dark soy sauce (1 tbsp.)
- Minced ginger (2 tsp.)
- Green onions (.25 cup)
- Salt (.5 tsp.)
- Sugar (2 tsp.)
- Sesame oil (1 tbsp.)

Ingredients - The Mayo:

- Gochujang (1 tbsp.)
- Mayonnaise (.25 cup)
- Sesame oil (1 tbsp.)
- Scallions (.25 cup - chopped)
- Sesame seeds (2 tsp.)
- *For Serving*: Hamburger buns (4)

Preparation Technique:

1. Combine the ground beef, garlic, ginger, gochujang, salt, sugar, sesame oil, soy sauce, and chopped onion. Let the mixture rest for 30 minutes or up to 24 hours in the refrigerator.
2. Shape the meat mixture into four rounded patties. Make a small impression in the middle to prevent the burgers from puffing into a dome-shape while cooking.
3. Set the fryer to 360° Fahrenheit for 10 minutes and arrange the patties in the Air Fryer basket (not touching).

4. Prepare the mayo. Whilst the patties are cooking, whisk and mix the mayonnaise, sesame oil, gochujang, sesame seeds, and scallions.
5. It's done when the center of the meat reaches 160° Fahrenheit. Place on the serving dish.
6. Serve the patties with hamburger buns and a serving of the delicious mayonnaise.

Beef Empanadas

Yields Provided: 4 Servings
Ingredients:
- Onion (1 small)
- Cloves of garlic (2)
- Olive oil (1 tbsp.)
- Ground beef (1 lb.)
- Empanada shells (1 pkg.)
- Green pepper (.5 of 1)
- Cumin (.5 tsp.)
- Tomato salsa (.25 cup)
- Egg yolk (1)
- Pepper and sea salt (to your liking)

Preparation Technique:
1. Peel and mince the garlic and onion. Deseed and dice the pepper.
2. Pour the oil to a skillet using the high-heat setting.
3. Fry the ground beef until browned. Drain the grease and add the onions and garlic. Cook for 4 minutes. Combine the remainder of fixings (omitting the milk, egg, and shells for now). Cook using the low setting for 10 minutes.
4. Make an egg wash with the yolk and milk.
5. Add the meat to half of the rolled dough brushing the edges with the wash. Fold it over and seal with a fork, brushing with the wash, and adding it to the basket.
6. Continue the process until all are done. Cook in the Air Fryer for 10 minutes at 350° Fahrenheit. Serve.

Beef Schnitzel

Yields Provided: 1 Serving
Ingredients:

- Olive oil (2 tbsp.)
- Thin beef schnitzel (1)
- Gluten-free breadcrumbs (.5 cup)
- Egg (1)

Preparation Technique:

1. Warm up the Air Fryer a couple of minutes (356° Fahrenheit).
2. Mix the breadcrumbs and oil in a shallow bowl. Whisk the egg in another mixing container.
3. Dip the beef into the egg, and then the breadcrumbs. Arrange in the basket of the Air Fryer.
4. Fry 12 minutes and serve.

Beef Steak Served Medium Rare

Yields Provided: 1 Serving
Ingredients:
- Beefsteak (1 - 1.5-inch thickness)
- Salt & Black pepper (to your liking)
- Spritz of olive oil cooking spray

Preparation Technique:
1. Set the Air Fryer at 350° Fahrenheit.
2. Spritz oil, salt, and pepper over the steak.
3. Place the beef on a baking tray. Cook for three minutes on each side.

Beef Stew

Yields Provided: 6 Servings
Ingredients:
- Butter (2 tsp.)
- Beef short ribs (10 oz.)
- Salt (.25 tsp.)
- Turmeric (1 tsp.)
- Chili flakes (.5 tsp.)
- Green pepper (1)
- Kale (4 oz.)
- Chicken stock (1 cup)
- Onion (.5 of 1)
- Green peas 4 oz.)

Preparation Technique:
1. Set the temperature of the Air Fryer at 360° Fahrenheit.
2. Measure the two teaspoons of butter to melt in the fryer basket. Add the ribs. Sprinkle with the salt, turmeric, and chili flakes. Set the timer for 15 minutes.
3. Remove the seeds and chop the kale and green pepper. Dice the onion.
4. When it's completed, pour in the stock, peppers, onions, peas and the peeled garlic clove.
5. Stir well and add the chopped kale. Set the timer for 8 more minutes.
6. Let the stew steep for a short while to blend the flavors before serving.

Black Peppercorns Meatloaf

Yields Provided: 4 Servings
Ingredients:
- Ground beef (4.5 lb.)
- Parsley (1 tbsp.)
- Basil (1 tbsp.)
- Oregano (1 tbsp.)
- Salt and pepper (to your liking)
- Large onion (1 diced)
- Worcestershire sauce (1 tsp.)
- Tomato ketchup (3 tbsp.)
- Breadcrumbs (if homemade - 1 slice of bread)

Preparation Technique:
1. Program the temperature setting to reach 356° Fahrenheit.
2. In a large mixing bowl, toss the beef, herbs, onion, Worcestershire sauce, and ketchup. Mix well for about 5 minutes. Mix in the breadcrumbs.
3. Add the meatloaf into the baking dish and arrange it in the Air Fryer basket. Cook for 25 minutes.

Carne Asada

Yields Provided: 4 Servings
Ingredients:
- Medium limes (2)
- Medium orange (1)
- Ancho chile powder (2 tsp.)
- Splenda (1 tsp.) or a substitute for 2 tsp. sugar
- Salt (1 tsp.)
- Cumin seeds (1 tsp.)
- Coriander seeds (1 tsp.)
- Cilantro (1 cup)
- Jalapeno - diced (1)
- Vinegar (2 tbsp.)
- Vegetable oil (2 tbsp.)
- Skirt steak (1.5 lb.)

Preparation Technique:
1. Peel the orange, and remove the seeds. Juice the limes.
2. Dice the jalapeno and toss all of the fixings into a blender, except the steak. Prepare until creamy.
3. Slice the steak into four pieces and add to a zipper-type bag. Marinate for a minimum of 30 minutes or up to one day in the fridge.
4. Set the Air Fryer temperature to 400° Fahrenheit.
5. Add the steaks into the basket and set the timer for 8 minutes. The internal temperature should reach 145° Fahrenheit.
6. When it's done, wait for 10 minutes to prevent toughness. Slice the meat against the grain.
7. Serve with your favorite side dish.

Cheeseburger Mini Sliders

Yields Provided: 3 Large Servings
Ingredients:
- Cheddar cheese (6 slices)
- Ground beef (1 lb.)
- Dinner rolls (6)
- Black pepper and Salt (to your liking)

Preparation Technique:
1. Set the temperature setting on the Air Fryer to 390° Fahrenheit.
2. Form 6 (2 .5 oz.) patties and season using the pepper and salt.
3. Arrange the burgers on the fryer basket for ten minutes.
4. Take them from the cooker and add the cheese. Return them to the Air Fryer for another minute until the cheese melts.

Cheeseburger Patties

Yields Provided: 6 Servings
Ingredients:
- Ground beef (1 lb.)
- Black pepper and salt (as desired)
- Cheddar cheese (6 slices)

Preparation Technique:
1. Set the temperature in the Air Fryer to 320° Fahrenheit.
2. Combine the ingredients and fully mix.
3. Shape into six burgers.
4. Air fry for ten minutes or as needed and serve.

Cheeseburgers Inside Out

Yields Provided: 4 Servings
Ingredients:
- Cheddar cheese (4 slices)
- Lean ground beef (.75 lb. or 12 oz.)
- Ketchup (4 tsp.)
- Minced onion (3 tbsp.)
- Salt & black pepper (as desired)
- Yellow mustard (2 tsp.)
- Dill pickle chips (8)

Preparation Technique:
1. Warm the Air Fryer until it reaches 370° Fahrenheit.
2. Dice the cheese into small pieces.
3. In a large mixing container, combine the ground beef, ketchup, pepper, salt, and mustard. Make four patties. Place two burgers, side by side.
4. Flatten the patty and add four pickle chips, and aa layer of cheese.
5. Smash a patty on top, pressing the meat together tightly to enclose all of the fixings.
6. Arrange the burgers in the basket and cook for twenty minutes. Turn them over after about 10 minutes.
7. Serve on a bun with tomato and lettuce.

Corned Beef

Servings Provided: 3
Ingredients:
- Onion (1)
- Water (1 cup)
- Minced beef (1 lb.)
- Black pepper (1 tsp.)
- Butter (1 tsp.)
- Cayenne pepper (.25 tsp.)
- Ground paprika (.5 tsp.)

Preparation Technique:
1. Warm the Air Fryer to reach 400° Fahrenheit.
2. Peel and finely slice the onion. Pour water into the tray and add the onion. Sprinkle with the spices. Stir and cook for four minutes.
3. Mince the garlic and add it to the mixture. Stir and add back to the Air Fryer. Continue cooking for seven minutes.
4. Carefully stir in the beef and cook for an additional eight minutes.
5. Remove from the fryer and add it to the plates for serving.

Country Fried Steak

Yields Provided: 1 Serving
Ingredients:
- Sirloin steak (1 - 6 oz.)
- Eggs (3)
- Panko (1 cup)
- Flour (1 cup)
- Pepper & salt (1 tsp. each)
- Garlic powder (1 tsp.)
- Onion powder (1 tsp.)
- Ground sausage (6 oz.)
- Pepper (1 tsp.)
- Flour (2 tbsp.)
- Milk (2 cups)

Preparation Technique:
1. Use a meat mallet to beat the steak until thin. Add the seasonings with the panko.
2. Dredge the beef through the flour, egg, and panko.
3. Arrange the prepared steak in the basket. Set the temperature to 370° Fahrenheit. Set the timer for 12 minutes. Remove the steak.
4. Prepare the gravy. Cook the sausage and drain on a few paper towels, saving two tablespoons in the pan. Blend in the flour and sausage. Mix well.
5. Pour in the milk and pepper, mixing until thickened. Fry for three more minutes before serving.

Herbed Shredded Beef

Yields Provided: 8 Servings
Ingredients:
- Thyme (1 tsp.)
- Salt (1 tsp.)
- Ground black pepper (1 tsp.)
- Mustard (1 tsp.)
- Dried dill (1 tsp.)
- Steak of choice (2 lb.)
- Butter (3 tbsp.)
- Chicken stock (4 cups)
- Peeled garlic clove (1)
- Bay leaf (1)
- Almond flour (1 tsp.)

Preparation Technique:
1. Set the Air Fryer in advance to reach 350° Fahrenheit.
2. Whisk the egg, baking powder, stevia, and butter.
3. Reserve one teaspoon of the almond flour and add the rest to the mixture. Knead until it's smooth - not sticky.
4. Cover the fryer basket with a layer of parchment paper. Add the prepared crust and flatten. Place the berries on top with a sprinkle of the almond flour.
5. Prepare in the Air Fryer for 20 minutes. Remove it when it's golden brown.
6. Chill and slice to serve with a delicious side salad.

Maggi Hamburgers

Yields Provided: 4 Servings
Ingredients:

- Maggi seasoning sauce (1 tsp.)
- Dried parsley (1 tsp.)
- Worcestershire sauce (1 tbsp.)
- Liquid smoke (1-2 drops)
- Dried oregano (.5 tsp.)
- Ground black pepper (.5 tsp.)
- Salt substitute (.5 tsp.)
- Onion powder (.5 tsp.)
- Garlic powder (.5 tsp.)
- 93% lean ground beef (1 lb.)

Preparation Technique:

1. Set the temperature in the Air Fryer to 350° Fahrenheit.
2. Combine all of the seasonings in a small dish and blend in the beef. Mix well until just combined.
3. Make four patties and arrange them on the tray together.
4. Cook for ten minutes – depending on the desired doneness (no need to flip). Serve when ready.

Quick & Easy Rib Steak

Yields Provided: 2 Servings
Ingredients:

- Steak rub - your preference (1 tbsp.)
- Rib steaks (2 lb.)
- Olive oil (1 tbsp.)

Preparation Technique:

1. Before it is time to cook, set the Air Fryer at 400° Fahrenheit.
2. Dust the steak using the oil and rub.
3. Place it in the basket to fry for 14 minutes, flipping after seven minutes.
4. Wait for at least 10 minutes before you slice to serve.

Roast Beef- Sandwich-Style

Yields Provided: 6 Servings

Ingredients:

- Garlic powder (.5 tsp.)
- Oregano (.5 tsp.)
- Dried thyme (1 tsp.)
- Olive oil (1 tbsp.)
- Round roast (2 lb.)

Preparation Technique:

1. Heat the Air Fryer to 330° Fahrenheit.
2. Combine the spices. Brush the oil over the beef, and rub it using the spice mixture.
3. Add to a baking dish and place it in the fryer basket for 30 minutes. Turn it over and continue cooking 25 more minutes.
4. Wait for a few minutes before slicing.
5. Serve on your choice of bread or eat it as it is.

Chapter 8: Other Delicious Meat Options

Cheesy Hot Dogs

Yields Provided: 2 Servings
Ingredients:
- Hot dogs (2)
- Hot dog buns (2)
- Grated cheese (2 tbsp.)

Preparation Technique:
1. Warm the Air Fryer for four minutes at 390° Fahrenheit.
2. Arrange the hot dogs in the fryer and cook for five minutes.
3. Place the hot dog on the bun and garnish with cheese.
4. Place in the fryer for about two minutes to melt the cheese and serve.

Delicious Stromboli

Yields Provided: 4 Servings

Ingredients:

- Refrigerated pizza crust - homemade or store-bought (12 oz.)
- Sliced cooked ham (.33 lb.)
- Roasted red bell peppers (3 oz.)
- Mozzarella shredded cheese (.75 cup)
- Shredded cheddar cheese (3 cups)
- Milk (1 tbsp.)
- Egg yolk (1)

Preparation Technique:

1. Warm up the Air Fryer at 360° Fahrenheit.
2. Roll the dough to reach a ¼-inch thickness.
3. Add the peppers, ham, and cheese on one side of the dough and fold to close.
4. Whisk the milk and eggs to make an egg wash, and brush the dough.
5. Place the stromboli in the basket and set the timer for 15 minutes.
6. Check it at 5-minute intervals - flipping the stromboli for thorough cooking.

Chapter 9: Veggies & Side Dishes

Asparagus & Smoked Cheese

Yields Provided: 4 Servings

Ingredients:
- Smoked – shredded gouda cheese (.25 cup)
- Italian seasoning (2 tbsp.)
- Parmesan cheese (.5 cup)
- Sea salt (.5 tsp.)
- Freshly cracked black pepper (.25 tsp.)
- Heavy cream (1 cup)
- Asparagus (1 lb.)

Preparation Technique:
1. Set the Air Fryer temperature at 400° Fahrenheit.
2. Use a sharp knife to discard the ¼-inch portion each asparagus.
3. Whisk the heavy cream, Italian seasoning, and parmesan.
4. Arrange the asparagus in a shallow dish and cover with the mixture.
5. Place in the basket of the fryer. Set the timer for 6 minutes.
6. Serve with the asparagus a sprinkle of cheese, pepper, and salt.

Avocado Fries

Yields Provided: 2 Servings
Ingredients:
- Large avocado (1)
- Breadcrumbs (.5 cup)
- Egg (1)
- Salt (.5 tsp.)

Preparation Technique:
1. Set the Air Fryer to 390° Fahrenheit. Peel, remove the pit and slice the avocado.
2. Prepare 2 shallow dishes, one with the breadcrumbs, and salt; and one with a whisked egg.
3. Dip the avocado into the egg – then the breadcrumbs.
4. Add to the fryer for 10 minutes.
5. Serve as a side dish or an appetizer.

Avocado & Bacon Fries

Yields Provided: 2 Servings
Ingredients:
- Egg (1)
- Almond flour (1 cup)
- Bacon – cooked – small bits (4 strips)
- Avocados (2 large)
- *For Frying*: Olive oil

Preparation Technique:
1. Warm the Air Fryer to 355° Fahrenheit.
2. Whisk the eggs in one container. Add the flour with the bacon in another.
3. Slice the avocado using lengthwise cuts. Dip into the eggs, then the flour mixture.
4. Drizzle oil in the fryer tray and cook for 10 minutes per side or until they're the way you like them.

Baked Potatoes

Yields Provided: 3 Servings
Ingredients:
- Russet or Idaho baking potatoes (3)
- Garlic (1 tbsp.)
- Salt(1 tbsp.)
- Parsley (1 tsp.)
- Olive oil (1-2 tbsp.)

Preparation Technique:
1. Rinse the potatoes and prick to make holes using a fork.
2. Oil and sprinkle the potatoes with the seasonings.
3. Add them to the Air Fryer basket and set the timer for 35-40 minutes.
4. Top it off using sour cream and fresh parsley.

Battered Baby Ears Of Corn

Yields Provided: 4 Servings
Ingredients:
- Carom seeds (.5 tsp.)
- Almond flour (1 cup)
- Chili powder (.25 tsp.)
- Garlic powder (1 tsp.)
- Boiled baby ears of corn (4)
- Baking soda (1 pinch)
- Salt (to your liking)

Preparation Technique:
1. Set the Air Fryer temperature at 350° Fahrenheit.
2. Sift or whisk the flour, salt, baking soda, garlic powder, chili powder, and carom seeds.
3. Pour a tiny amount of water into a bowl to make a batter. Dip the boiled corn in the mixture and arrange it in a foil-lined fryer basket. Set a timer for ten minutes.
4. Serve with your favorite entrée.

Blossoming Onions

Yields Provided: 4 Servings

Ingredients:
- Small onions (4)
- Dollops of butter (4)
- Olive oil (1 tbsp.)

Preparation Technique:
1. Peel the skin from the onion and remove the top and bottom to create flat ends.
2. Soak the onions in salted water for four hours to remove the harshness.
3. Slice the onion as far down as you can without severing the onion body. Cut four times - making eight segments.
4. Preheat the fryer to 350° Fahrenheit.
5. Toss the prepared onions into the fryer basket. Drizzle with oil, adding a dollop of butter to each one.
6. Cook in the fryer until the outside is dark (30 min.).
7. *Note*: 4 dollops = 4 heaping tbsp.

Brussels Sprouts

Yields Provided: 4-5 Servings or Approx. 1 pound
Ingredients:
- Olive oil (5 tbsp.)
- Fresh brussels sprouts (1 lb.)
- Kosher salt (.5 tsp.)

Preparation Technique:
1. Prep the vegetables. Trim the stems and discard any damaged outer leaves. Cut into halves, rinse, and pat dry. Toss with the oil and salt.
2. Set the fryer temperature ahead of time to 390° Fahrenheit.
3. Toss the sprouts into the basket and air-fry for 15 minutes.
4. Shake the basket to ensure even browning.

Buffalo Cauliflower

Yields Provided: 4 Servings

Ingredients:
- Breadcrumbs (1 cup)
- Cauliflower florets (4 cups)
- Buffalo sauce (.25 cup)
- Melted butter (.25 cup)
- *For the Dip*: Your favorite dressing

Preparation Technique:
1. Melt the butter in a microwaveable dish. Whisk in the buffalo sauce.
2. Dip the florets in the butter mixture. Use the stem as a handle; holding it over a cup and let the excess drip away.
3. Run the floret through the breadcrumbs. Drop them into the fryer. Air-fry for 14 to 17 minutes at 350° Fahrenheit. (The unit *will not* need to preheat since it is calculated into the time.)
4. Shake the basket several times during the cooking process. Enjoy alongside your favorite dip, making sure to eat it right away because the crunchiness goes away quickly.
5. *Cooking Note:* Reheat in the oven. Don't use the microwave or it will be mushy.

Butternut Squash

Yields Provided: 4 Servings
Ingredients:
- Butternut squash (1 medium)
- Cumin seeds (2 tsp.)
- Chili flakes (1 pinch)
- Salt & black pepper (as desired)
- Coriander (1 bunch)
- Pine nuts (.25 cup)
- Olive oil (1 tbsp.)
- Greek yogurt (.66 cup)

Preparation Technique:
1. Set the Air Fryer temperature in advance to 380° Fahrenheit.
2. Cube the squash and toss using the spices and oil in a baking pan.
3. Add them to the fryer for 20 minutes.
4. Toast the pine nuts. Serve with a portion of yogurt and a sprinkle of coriander to top it off.

Carrots Zucchini & Yellow Squash

Yields Provided: 4 Servings
Ingredients:
- Diced carrots (.5 lb.)
- Olive oil - divided (6 tsp.)
- Lime wedges (1)
- Zucchini – .75-inch semi-circles (1 lb.)
- Yellow squash (1 lb.)
- Chopped tarragon leaves (1 tbsp.)
- Sea salt (1 tsp.)
- White pepper (.5 tsp.)

Preparation Technique:
1. Set the Air Fryer temperature to 400° Fahrenheit.
2. Trim the squash and zucchini.
3. Dice the carrots into a bowl with 2 teaspoons of oil. Toss and add them to the fryer basket. Set the timer for 5 minutes.
4. Place the squash and zucchini in the bowl with the rest of the oil, salt, and pepper.
5. When the carrots are done, mix in the rest of the fixings. Cook for 30 minutes. Stir occasionally and garnish using the tarragon and lime wedges.

Cauliflower Curried Florets

Yields Provided: 4 Servings
Ingredients:

- Boiling water (1 cup)
- Golden raisins/Sultanas (.25 cup)
- Pine nuts (.25 cup)
- Olive oil (.5 cup)
- Salt (.25 tsp.)
- Curry powder (1 tbsp.)
- Cauliflower (1 head – small florets)

Preparation Technique:

1. Measure and toss the raisins into a cup of boiling water to plump.
2. Warm the Air Fryer temperature at 350° Fahrenheit.
3. Toast the nuts in the fryer with the oil for about a minute.
4. Toss the florets with the curry powder and salt in a bowl. Add to the Air Fryer. Set the timer for 10 minutes. Drain and toss all of the fixings well before serving.

Charred Shishito Peppers

Yields Provided: 4 Servings
Ingredients:
- Olive oil (1 tsp.)
- Juiced lemon (1)
- Shishito peppers (20)
- Sea salt (as desired)

Preparation Technique:
1. Heat the Air Fryer to reach 390° Fahrenheit.
2. Toss the peppers in with the oil and salt. Add them to the basket and air-fry for five minutes.
3. Serve on a platter with a squeeze of lemon.

Cheesy Broccoli & Olives

Yields Provided: 2-4 Servings
Ingredients:

- Broccoli crowns (2 lb.)
- Olive oil (2 tbsp.)
- Kosher salt (1 tsp.)
- Black pepper (.5 tsp.)
- Grated lemon zest (2 tsp.)
- Kalamata olives (.33 cup)
- Shaved parmesan cheese (.25 cup)

Preparation Technique:

1. Remove the stems from the broccoli and slice them into 1 to 1.5-inch florets. Remove the pit and slice the olives in half.
2. Over the high-heat setting, fill a medium pan with 6 cups of water. Wait for it to boil. Toss in the florets and cook for three to four minutes. Remove and drain on a layer of paper towels. Add the pepper, salt, and oil.
3. Warm the Air Fryer to reach 400° Fahrenheit. Toss the prepared broccoli into the basket, close the drawer, and click the timer for 15 minutes. Flip after about seven minutes for even browning.
4. When done, place the broccoli in the bowl. Garnish with lemon zest, olives, and cheese. Enjoy immediately.

Chicken Fried Rice

Yields Provided: 5-6 Servings
Ingredients:
- Frozen carrots and peas (1 cup)
- Cold cooked white rice (3 cups)
- Vegetable oil (1 tbsp.)
- Soy sauce (6 tbsp.)
- Packed cooked chicken (1 cup)
- Diced onion (.5 cup)
- *Also Needed:* 7 by 2-inch cake pan

Preparation Technique:
1. Set the Air Fryer at 360° Fahrenheit.
2. Cook and dice the chicken. Prepare the rice. Dice the onion.
3. Add the chilled white rice, soy sauce, and oil into a mixing bowl. Stir well.
4. Toss in the onion, chicken, peas, and carrots. Combine the fixings in the Air Fryer and set the timer for 20 minutes.
5. Serve as a side with your favorite meal or enjoy it alone.

Crispy 'N' Spicy Cauliflower

Yields Provided: 4 Servings
Ingredients:
- Hot sauce (.25 cup)
- Melted butter (.25 cup)
- Cauliflower florets (4 cups)
- Breadcrumbs (1 cup)

Preparation Technique:
1. Set the fryer temperature to 350° Fahrenheit.
2. Whisk the hot sauce and melted butter in a mixing container.
3. Prepare the florets and toss them into the mixture.
4. Coat them using the breadcrumbs and place them in the basket of the Air Fryer. Cook for 15 minutes, shaking several times.
5. Serve with a favorite dip.

Crispy Onion Rings

Yields Provided: 2 Servings
Ingredients:
- Coconut flour (2 tbsp.)
- Grated parmesan cheese (2 tbsp.)
- Egg (1)
- Large onion (1 in ringlets)
- Garlic powder (1 pinch)
- Pepper and salt (as desired)
- Olive oil (.25 cup)

Preparation Technique:
1. Whisk the flour, spices, and grated cheese.
2. Set the Air Fryer at 400° Fahrenheit.
3. Whisk the eggs in a separate mixing container and add the onion rings. Soak a minute or so, and dip into the flour mixture.
4. Place in the Air Fryer basket, setting the timer for 6 minutes per side.
5. Serve as a quick snack or favorite side dish.

Crunchy Black-Eyed Peas

Yields Provided: 6 Servings
Ingredients:

- Black-eyed peas (15 oz. can)
- Salt (.25 tsp.)
- Chipotle chili powder (.125 tsp.)
- Black pepper (.125 tsp.)
- Chili powder (.5 tsp.)

Preparation Technique:

1. Use cold tap water to thoroughly rinse the beans. Set aside for now.
2. Preheat the Air Fryer to 360° Fahrenheit.
3. Whisk the spices and mix with the peas. Stir well.
4. Toss into the fryer basket and cook for ten minutes.
5. Serve with your favorite dinner meal.

Cumin & Chili Squash

Yields Provided: 2 Servings
Ingredients:
- Medium butternut squash (1)
- Greek yogurt (.66 cup)
- Coriander (1 bunch)
- Pine nuts (.25 cup)
- Cumin seeds (2 tsp.)
- Chili flakes (1 pinch)
- Black pepper and salt (to your liking)
- Olive oil (1 tbsp.)

Preparation Technique:
1. Set the Air Fryer temperature setting at 380°F.
2. Dice the squash, and combine it with the oil and spices in a baking pan.
3. Add them to the fryer for 20 minutes.
4. Toast the pine nuts and serve alongside the yogurt and a sprinkle of coriander to top it off.

Daikon Fries

Yields Provided: 2 Servings
Ingredients:

- Daikon (1)
- Salt and pepper (to your liking)
- Melted coconut oil (.25 cup)

Preparation Technique:

1. Peel and slice the daikon into fries.
2. Set the Air Fryer temperature to 450° Fahrenheit.
3. Combine the ingredients and toss the fries into the basket.
4. Set the timer for 15 minutes.
5. Shake about halfway through the cycle. Serve while hot.

Delicious Tofu

Yields Provided: 4 Servings

Ingredients:

- Sesame oil (2 tbsp.)
- Cornstarch (1 tbsp.)
- Tofu (1 block tofu – 1-inch cubes)
- Rice vinegar (1 tsp.)
- Soy sauce (2 tbsp.)

Preparation Technique:

1. Set the fryer ahead of time to reach 370° Fahrenheit.
2. Mix the oil, vinegar, tofu, and soy sauce substitute of your choice. Toss well and set aside.
3. Toss the cornstarch in a dish and cover the tofu.
4. Place in the Air Fryer basket for 20 minutes. Shake a few times during the cycle. Serve.

Feta Grilled Corn

Yields Provided: 2 Servings
Ingredients:
- Corn-on-the-cobs (2 whole)
- Olive oil (1 tsp.)
- Paprika (2 tsp.)
- Grated feta cheese (.5 cup)

Preparation Technique:
1. Remove the husks and silks. Generously grease the corn with the oil and give it a sprinkle of the paprika.
2. Set the Air Fryer temperature at 392° Fahrenheit.
3. Grill for 15 minutes and serve with the cheese.

Garlic & Thyme Tomatoes

Yields Provided: 4 Servings
Ingredients:
- Olive oil (1 tbsp.)
- Roma tomatoes (4)
- Clove of garlic (1)
- Dried thyme (.5 tsp.)
- Freshly ground black pepper & salt (to taste)

Preparation Technique:
1. Set the temperature of the Air Fryer to 390° Fahrenheit.
2. Mince the garlic clove. Slice the tomatoes and remove the pithy parts and seeds. Toss them into a mixing container along with the pepper, salt, thyme, garlic, and olive oil.
3. Arrange them in the fryer with the cut side up. Set a timer for 15 minutes.
4. Cool for a few minutes. Add on top of poultry, fish, or pasta.

Grilled Tomatoes

Yields Provided: 2 Servings
Ingredients:
- Tomatoes (2)
- Black pepper & Herbs of choice (sage, oregano, basil, etc.)
- Cooking oil spray (as needed)

Preparation Technique:
1. Preheat the fryer to 320° Fahrenheit.
2. Wash and slice the tomatoes into halves. Spray each one lightly using a spritz of cooking oil spray. Place them cut-side facing upwards. Sprinkle using your favorite spices—fresh or dried - such as pepper, sage, rosemary, basil, oregano, and any others of your choice.
3. Arrange them in the basket and air-fry for 20 minutes or until they're the way you like them. Enjoy if they are ready—if not—cook for a few more minutes.

Honey Roasted Carrots

Yields Provided: 4 Servings

Ingredients:

- Carrots - baby or regular (3 cups)
- Honey (1 tbsp.)
- Olive oil (1 tbsp.)
- Pepper and salt (as desired)

Preparation Technique:

1. Warm the fryer to reach 392° Fahrenheit. Dice the carrots into small chunks.
2. Combine the honey, oil, and carrots in a mixing bowl, coating well.
3. Sprinkle with some pepper and salt.
4. Put the carrots into the Air Fryer and set the timer for 12 minutes.

Lemon - Green Beans

Yields Provided: 4 Servings
Ingredients:
- Lemon (1)
- Green beans (1 lb.)
- Olive oil (.25 tsp.)
- Black pepper and sea salt (to your liking)

Preparation Technique:
1. Warm the Air Fryer (400° Fahrenheit).
2. Rinse, and dump the green beans into the fryer basket with a squeeze of lemon along with the oil, salt, and pepper.
3. Toss well and set the timer for 12 minutes. Serve right away.

Mediterranean Veggies

Yields Provided: 4 Servings
Ingredients:
- Cherry tomatoes (.25 cup)
- Medium carrot (1)
- Green pepper (1
- Large parsnip (1)
- Large cucumber (1)
- Garlic puree (2 tbsp.)
- Honey (2 tbsp.)
- Olive oil (6 tbsp.)
- Mixed herbs (1 tsp.)
- Pepper & salt (to your liking)

Preparation Technique:
1. Set the Air Fryer at 356° Fahrenheit.
2. Chop the cucumber and green pepper. Toss them into the Air Fryer.
3. Peel and dice the carrot and parsnip, adding the whole cherry tomatoes. Drizzle with three tbsp. of oil. Set the timer for 15 minutes.
4. Mix the rest of the fixings in an Air Fryer - safe baking dish.
5. Add the veggies to the marinade and shake well. Give it a sprinkle of pepper and salt and cook at 392° Fahrenheit for another five minutes.
6. *Note*: You can substitute and experiment with different veggies, but don't use the cucumber and cauliflower in the same dish. Together, they produce too much liquid.
7. For variety, serve with a portion of honey and sweet potatoes to the mixture.

Mushroom Melt

Yields Provided: 10 loaded mushrooms
Ingredients:
- Button mushrooms (10)
- Italian dried mixed herbs
- Salt and pepper
- Mozzarella cheese
- Cheddar cheese
- *Optional Garnish*: Dried dill

Preparation Technique:
1. Rinse the mushrooms, remove the stems, and drain in a colander.
2. Flavor with a pinch of chosen herbs, black pepper, salt, and olive oil.
3. Warm the Air Fryer ahead of time to reach 356° Fahrenheit. (3-5 min.)
4. Arrange the mushrooms in the basket with the hollow section facing you. Sprinkle the cheese on top of each of the caps.
5. Place the mushrooms in the cooker for 7-8 minutes.
6. Serve hot with a drizzle of basil or other tasty herbs.

Pesto & Feta Baked Tomatoes

Yields Provided: 4 Servings

Ingredients - The Pesto:
- Toasted pine nuts (3 tbsp.)
- Garlic (1 toasted clove)
- Grated parmesan cheese (.5 cup) t
- Freshly chopped mix – basil & parsley (.5 cup)
- Olive oil (1 tbsp.)
- Salt (1 pinch)

Ingredients - Tomatoes & Feta:
- Red onion (.5 cup)
- Feta cheese (8 oz.)
- Heirloom tomatoes (2)
- Olive oil (1 tbsp.)
- Salt (1 pinch)

Preparation Technique:
1. Slice the red onion very thin. Also, cut the cheese and tomatoes into ½-inch slices.
2. Prepare the pesto – omit the salt and oil- using a food processor. Once a thick paste is formed; add the salt, tomatoes, feta, and onion.
3. Set the Air Fryer at 350° Fahrenheit.
4. Arrange the mixture in the food tray and set the timer for 14 minutes.
5. Serve when ready.

Roasted Cauliflower with Nuts & Raisins

Yields Provided: 4 Servings
Ingredients:
- Olive oil (3.5 oz./.33 cup + 2 tbsp.)
- Cauliflower florets (1 small head)
- Toasted pine nuts (2 tbsp.)
- Raisins (2 tbsp.)
- Salt (.5 tsp.)
- Curry powder (1 tsp.)

Preparation Technique:
1. Soak the raisins in a dish of boiling water and drain.
2. Warm up the fryer to 320° Fahrenheit (2 min.).
3. Combine the fixings in a bowl and add them to the basket.
4. Set the timer for 15 minutes and serve.

Semolina Veggie Cutlets

Yields Provided: 2 Servings
Ingredients:
- Olive oil – for frying
- Semolina (1 cup)
- Salt & Pepper (to your liking)
- Veggies of choice - ex. carrots, cauliflower, peas, green beans, etc. (1.5 cups total)
- Milk (5 cups)

Preparation Technique:
1. Warm the milk in a saucepan (med. heat). When hot, add the vegetables, pepper, and salt. Set the timer for 3 minutes.
2. Mix in the semolina and fry for another 10 minutes.
3. Prepare a baking sheet with a sheet of parchment baking paper. Spread the mixture over the pan to chill in the fridge for a minimum of four hours.
4. Set the Air Fryer temperature to 350° Fahrenheit.
5. Remove the mixture from the fridge and slice into cutlets. Brush with oil and bake for 10 minutes.
6. Serve with a portion of hot sauce.

Tawa Vegetables

Yields Provided: 4 Servings
Ingredients:
- Potato (.25 cup)
- Okra (.25 cup)
- Taro root (.25 cup)
- Eggplant (.25 cup)
- Garam masala (2 tsp.)
- Red chili powder (1 tsp.)
- Amchur powder (1 tsp.)
- Salt (as desired)
- *For Brushing*: Olive oil

Preparation Technique:
1. Set the Air Fryer at 390° Fahrenheit.
2. Slice the taro root and potatoes into fries, and soak in salted water for about ten minutes.
3. Slice the eggplant and okra into four segments.
4. Rinse the potatoes and taro root; pat dry. Combine with the spices, okra, and eggplant.
5. Brush the pan with oil and set the timer for ten minutes. Lower the heat setting to 355° Fahrenheit and cook for an additional 15 minutes.
6. Serve and enjoy the veggies any way you choose.

Zucchini Fries

Yields Provided: 2 Servings
Ingredients:

- Large zucchini (1)
- Eggs (2)
- Flour (.5 cup)
- Olive oil
- Salt and pepper (as desired)

Preparation Steps:

1. Set the Air Fryer temperature (400° Fahrenheit.)
2. Slice the zucchini into fry sticks and shake with pepper and salt.
3. Coat the fries with the flour then the egg (whisked in a bowl).
4. Lightly spray the fries with cooking oil spray and place them in the basket.
5. Set the timer for 6 minutes on each side.
6. Serve with your favorite entrée or as a snack.

Chapter 10: Delicious Bread Options

Air Bread & Egg Butter

Air Bread
Yields Provided: 19 Servings
Ingredients:

- Eggs (3)
- Baking powder (1 tsp.)
- Almond flour (1 cup)
- Sea salt (.25 tsp.)
- Unchilled butter (.25 cup)

Preparation Technique:

1. Program the Air Fryer to reach 350° Fahrenheit.
2. Soften the butter to room temperature. Whisk the eggs with a hand mixer. Combine and add the rest of the recipe components to make the dough.
3. Knead the dough and cover with a clean kitchen towel for about ten minutes.
4. Air fry the bread for 15 minutes.
5. Remove the bread and cool on a wooden cutting board.
6. Slice and serve.

Egg Butter
Yields Provided: 4 Servings
Ingredients:

- Eggs (4)
- Salt (1 tsp.)

- Butter (4 tbsp.)

Preparation Technique:
1. Warm the Air Fryer to reach 320° Fahrenheit.
2. Cover the Air Fryer basket with foil and add the eggs. Cook for 17 minutes. Transfer to an ice-cold water bath to chill.
3. Peel and chop the eggs and combine with the rest of the ingredients. Mix well until it's smooth.
4. Serve with the *Air Fried Bread.*

Bread Rolls with Potato Stuffing

Yields Provided: 4 Servings
Ingredients:
- Bread - white part only (8 slices)
- Potatoes (5 large)
- Finely chopped coriander (1 small bunch)
- Seeded and finely chopped green chilies (2)
- Turmeric (.5 tsp.)
- Curry leaf sprigs (2)
- Mustard seeds (.5 tsp.)
- Finely chopped small onions (2)
- Oil - frying and brushing (2 tbsp.)
- Salt (as desired)

Preparation Technique:
1. Warm up the Air Fryer to 392° Fahrenheit. Use a sharp knife to remove the edges of the bread.
2. Peel the potatoes, and boil. Mash the potatoes using 1 tsp. of salt.
3. Meanwhile, on the stovetop, prepare a skillet using 1 tsp. of oil. Toss in the mustard seeds and onions. When the seeds sputter, continue frying until they become translucent. Toss in the curry and turmeric.
4. Fry the mixture a few seconds and add the mashed potatoes. Mix well and let it cool. Shape eight portions of the dough into an oval shape. Set them aside for now.
5. Wet the bread with water and press it in your palm to remove the excess water. Place the oval potato into the bread and roll it around the potato mixture. Be sure they are completely sealed.
6. Brush the potato rolls with oil and set aside.
7. Set the timer for 12-13 minutes. Cook until crispy and browned.

Buttermilk Biscuits

Yields Provided: 2 Servings

Ingredients:
- Cake flour (.5 cup)
- Granulated sugar (1 tsp.)
- Baking powder (.5 tsp.)
- Salt (.75 tsp.)
- Baking soda (.25 tsp.)
- All-purpose flour (1.25 cups + more for countertop dusting)
- Buttermilk (.75 tsp.)
- Unsalted cold butter (4 tbsp. cut into cubes + melt 1 tbsp.)

Optional for Serving:
- Honey/preserves
- Butter

Preparation Technique:
1. Program the Air Fryer to 400° Fahrenheit.
2. Whisk or sift the all-purpose flour, baking soda, sugar, cake flour, and salt in a medium mixing dish.
3. Sprinkle flour on the countertop surface. Press the dough into about a ½-inch thickness (8-inches in diameter).
4. Cut the dough into biscuits. Dip the tip of the cutter with the flour making a swift cut. Don't twist the dough because it could prevent it from rising.
5. Arrange the biscuits in a pan. Brush them using the melted butter.
6. Place the dough in the basket of the fryer and set the timer for eight minutes. Serve with honey or your favorite preserves, jam, or jelly.

Cheesy Garlic Bread

Yields Provided: 3-4 Servings
Ingredients:
- Bread slices (5 rounds)
- Sun-dried tomato pesto (5 tsp.)
- Garlic cloves (3)
- Melted butter (4 tbsp.)
- Grated Mozzarella cheese (1 cup)

Garnish Options:
- Chili flakes
- Chopped basil leaves
- Oregano

Preparation Technique:
1. Warm the Air Fryer to reach 356° Fahrenheit.
2. Slice the bread loaf into five thick slices.
3. Spread the butter, pesto, and cheese onto the bread.
4. Put the slices in the Air Fryer for 6-8 minutes.
5. Garnish with your choice of toppings.
6. _Note_: Round or baguette bread was used for this recipe. It's recommended to add the finely chopped garlic cloves to the melted butter ahead of time for the best results.

Garlic Knots

Yields Provided: 4 Servings

Ingredients:
- Frozen pizza crust dough (1 lb.)
- Garlic powder (1 tbsp.)
- Grated Parmesan cheese (1 tbsp.)
- Freshly chopped parsley (1 tbsp.)
- Sea salt (1 tsp.)
- Marinara sauce (as desired)

Preparation Technique:
1. Set the Air Fryer at 360° Fahrenheit.
2. Roll out the dough until it is about 1.5 to 2-inches thick. Slice it approximately .75-inches apart—lengthwise.
3. Roll the dough and make it into knots.
4. Add the cheese, oil, and spices in a bowl, and roll each knot in the mixture before placing it into the fryer basket.
5. Set the timer for 12 minutes and flip the knots halfway through the cooking process (@ 6 minutes).
6. Serve with a dish of marinara sauce.

Chapter 11: Appetizers & Salty Snacks

Bacon & Cream Cheese Stuffed Jalapeno Poppers

Yields Provided: 5 Servings

Ingredients:
- Unchilled cream cheese – reduced-fat (6 oz.)
- Shredded cheddar cheese (.25 cup)
- Fresh jalapenos (10 oz.)
- Bacon (2 slices)

Preparation Technique:
1. Slice the jalapenos vertically into halves. Cut the seeds out of the jalapeno, saving a few if you like it hot. Prepare the bacon and crumble.
2. Place the cream cheese in a mixing container. Soften in the microwave for 15 seconds or leave it out for about 30 minutes on the countertop for spreadability.
3. Combine the fixings in a bowl. Add the seeds and stuff the hulls with the mixture.
4. Add the poppers into the Air Fryer and lightly spray with a spritz of cooking oil spray.
5. Close the fryer and set the timer for 5 minutes. Remove and cool slightly before serving.
6. *Note*: Cook about 3 more minutes if you like them crunchy.

Bacon Bacon-Wrapped Chicken

Yields Provided: 3 Servings
Ingredients:
- Chicken (1 breast)
- Soft garlic cheese (1 tbsp.)
- Unsmoked bacon (6 strips)

Preparation Technique:
1. Slice the chicken into six pieces.
2. Spread the garlic cheese over each bacon strip and add a piece of chicken to each one. Roll and secure using a toothpick.
3. Warm the Air Fryer in advance for 2-3 minutes to reach 390° Fahrenheit.
4. Add the wraps and set a timer for 15 minutes.

Bacon-Wrapped Shrimp

Yields Provided: 4 Servings
Ingredients:
- Bacon slices (1 lb.)
- Peeled prawns (1 lb.)

Preparation Technique:
1. Heat the Air Fryer ahead of baking time to reach 390° Fahrenheit.
2. Wrap a bacon slice around each shrimp and add to the fryer basket
3. Set the timer for five minutes and serve.

Bacon-Wrapped Tater Tots

Yields Provided: 4 Servings

Ingredients:
- Sour cream (3 tbsp.)
- Sliced bacon (1 lb.)
- Crispy tater tots (1 large bag)
- Scallions (4)
- Shredded cheddar cheese (.5 cup)

Preparation Technique:
1. Set the Air Fryer temperature at 400° Fahrenheit.
2. Wrap each of the tots in bacon. Arrange them in the fryer basket. Don't overcrowd; keep them in a single layer.
3. Set the fryer timer for 8 minutes.
4. Serve with the scallions, cheese, and a dash of sour cream.

Beef Roll-Ups

Yields Provided: 4 Servings
Ingredients:
- Beef flank steak (2 lb.)
- Pesto (3 tbsp.)
- Fresh baby spinach (.75 cup)
- Roasted red bell peppers (3 oz.)
- Provolone cheese (6 slices)
- Pepper & sea salt (as desired)

Preparation Technique:
1. Heat the Air Fryer to 400° Fahrenheit.
2. Slice the steak open (not all the way through) to spread the pesto over the meat.
3. Layer the peppers, cheese, and spinach (about ¾ of the way into the meat).
4. Roll it up with toothpicks. Give it a sprinkle of pepper and salt.
5. Set the timer for 4 minutes – rotating halfway through the cycle.
6. When it's done, wait for about 10 minutes before slicing to serve.

Beef & Bacon Taco Rolls

Yields Provided: 2 Servings
Ingredients:
- Ground beef (2 cups)
- Bacon bits (.5 cup)
- Tomato salsa (1 cup)
- Turmeric coconut wraps/your choice (4)
- Shredded Monterey Jack Cheese (1 cup)
- *To Your Liking - The Spices:*
    - Garlic powder
    - Chili powder
    - Black pepper

Preparation Technique:
1. Warm the fryer to reach 390° Fahrenheit.
2. Add all of the spice fixings together and toss with the beef.
3. Prepare and roll the wraps and place in the Air Fryer.
4. Set the timer for 15 minutes and serve.

Chicken Kabobs

Yields Provided: 2 Servings
Ingredients:
- Bell peppers – multi colors of your choice (3)
- Mushrooms (6)
- Soy sauce (.33 cup)
- Honey (.33 cup)
- Pepper and salt (as desired)
- Sesame seeds
- Chicken breasts (2)
- Cooking oil spray (as needed)

Preparation Technique:
1. Dice the chicken and peppers. Chop the mushrooms into halves. Give the chicken a couple of squirts of oil and a pinch of salt and pepper.
2. Combine the soy and honey – mixing well. Add sesame seeds and stir.
3. Insert the peppers, chicken, and mushroom bits onto a skewer.
4. Set the temperature of the Air Fryer to 338° Fahrenheit.
5. Cover the kabobs with the sauce and arrange them in the fryer basket.
6. Set the timer for 15-20 minutes and serve.

Crispy Gnocchi

Yields Provided: 4 Servings

Ingredients:
- Frozen gnocchi (12 oz.)
- Vegetable/olive oil (1-2 tbsp. or as needed)
- Parmesan cheese (3 tbsp. grated)
- *For Dipping:* Marinara sauce

Preparation Technique:
1. Set the Air Fryer temp to 350° Fahrenheit for one to two minutes.
2. Add the gnocchi into a bowl and toss it with oil (not coconut oil).
3. Toss the gnocchi in the fryer and fry for 8 to 10 minutes until they're starting to turn golden brown. Toss the fixings in the basket every few minutes to allow even cooking.
4. Remove the gnocchi from the Air Fryer and place it on a serving tray.
5. Lightly mist the tops with a spritz of oil if desired and a sprinkle of parmesan cheese.
6. Serve immediately with marinara on the side as a dipping sauce.

Mac "N" Cheese Balls

Yields Provided: 2 Servings
Ingredients:
- Macaroni and cheese (2 cups) or (.33 cup) Shredded cheddar cheese
- Eggs (3)
- Milk (2 cups)
- White flour (.75 cup)
- Plain breadcrumbs (1 cup)

Preparation Technique:
1. Set the temperature of the Air Fryer to 360° Fahrenheit.
2. Combine the leftovers with the shredded cheese.
3. Place the breadcrumbs into a dish.
4. Measure the flour into another bowl.
5. Combine the milk and eggs.
6. Prepare a small-sized ball from the macaroni and cheese.
7. Roll the balls in the flour, eggs, and lastly the breadcrumbs.
8. Place the balls in the fryer basket. Select the chicken icon.
9. Set the timer for 10 minutes – rotating halfway through the cooking cycle. Serve as a snack or delicious side dish.

Meatballs For The Party

Yields Provided: 24 Servings

Ingredients:
- Worcestershire sauce (2.5 tbsp.)
- Ground beef (1 lb.)
- Tabasco sauce (1 tbsp.)
- Lemon juice (1 tbsp.)
- Tomato ketchup (.75 cup)
- Vinegar (.25 cup)
- Dry mustard (.5 tsp.)
- Brown sugar (.5 cup)
- Crushed gingersnaps (3)

Preparation Technique:
1. Combine all of the seasonings in a large mixing container—blending well.
2. Mix the beef and continue churning the ingredients.
3. Make the balls and arrange them in the Air Fryer.
4. Cook on 375° Fahrenheit for 15 minutes. They're ready when the center is done. Place them on toothpicks before serving.

Mini Bacon-Wrapped Burritos (Vegan)

Yields Provided: 4 Servings
Ingredients:
- Water (1-2 tbsp.)
- Tofu Scramble or Vegan Egg (2 servings)
- Tamari (2-3 tbsp.)
- Cashew butter (2 tbsp.)
- Liquid smoke (1-2 tbsp.)
- Rice paper (4 pieces)

Ingredients - Vegetable Add-Ins:
- Roasted red pepper (8 strips)
- Sweet potato roasted cubes (.33 cup)
- Sautéed tree broccoli (1 small)
- Greens (1 small handful)
- Fresh asparagus (6-8 stalks)
- *Note*: You can add greens including kale, spinach, etc.

Preparation Technique:
1. Preheat the Air Fryer to 350° Fahrenheit.
2. Prepare a baking pan with parchment baking paper to fit inside the fryer.
3. Whisk the cashew butter, water, tamari, and liquid smoke. Set it aside for now.
4. *Prepare the Filling*: Hold a rice paper under cold running water to get both sides wet. Place on the plate to fill.
5. Start by filling the fixings –just off from the center– leaving the sides of the paper open.
6. Fold in two of the sides to make the burrito. Seal and dip each one in the liquid smoke mixture–coating completely.
7. Cook until crispy (8-10 min.). Serve when ready.

Mini Quiche Wedges

Yields Provided: 9 Servings

Ingredients:
- Homemade pizza crust or store-bought (3.5 oz.)
- Egg (1)
- Grated cheese (1.4 oz.)
- Oil (.5 tbsp.)
- Whipping cream (3 tbsp.)
- Fresh ground pepper & salt (as desired)
- Small pie molds (2)

Preparation Technique:
1. Warm the Air Fryer to reach 392° Fahrenheit before it's frying time.
2. Coat the molds using a spritz of cooking oil spray to grease the molds. Prepare by pressing the dough in and around the edges.
3. Whisk the cream, egg, cheese, pepper, and salt. Add to the prepared molds and place them in the basket. Set the timer for 12 minutes. Bake the second one using the same process.
4. When ready, transfer from the molds. Slice each of the quiches into six wedges. Serve at room temperature or warm.

Mozzarella Sticks

Yields Provided: 4 Servings
Ingredients:
- Eggs (2)
- Mozzarella cheese (1 lb./1 block)
- Plain breadcrumbs (1 cup)
- White flour (.25 cup)
- Nonfat milk (3 tbsp.)

Preparation Technique:
1. Set the temperature of the Air Fryer to 400° Fahrenheit.
2. Slice the cheese into ½-inch by 3-inch sticks.
3. Whisk the milk and eggs together in one bowl, with the oil and breadcrumbs in individual dishes as well.
4. Dredge the sliced cheese through the oil, egg, and breadcrumbs.
5. Place the sticks onto a bread tray and put them in the freezer compartment for about an hour or two.
6. Arrange them in small increments into the fryer basket. Cook for 12 minutes.

Mozzarella Turkey Rolls

Yields Provided: 4 Servings

Ingredients:
- Sliced tomato (1)
- Turkey breast (4 slices)
- Freshly chopped basil (.5 cup)
- Sliced mozzarella (1 cup)
- Chive shoots (4 for tying)

Preparation Technique:
1. Set the Air Fryer temperature to 390° Fahrenheit.
2. Add a slice of turkey, cheese, tomato, and basil.
3. Roll up each one and tie them with the chive shoot.
4. Arrange in the fryer for 10 minutes. Prepare and serve warm.

Pigs In A Blanket

Yields Provided: 4 Servings
Ingredients:

- Crescent rolls (8 oz. can)
- Cocktail wieners (12 oz. pkg.)

Preparation Technique:

1. Set the Air Fryer to 330° Fahrenheit.
2. Place the franks in paper towels to drain thoroughly. Slice the dough into strips of about 1.5 x 1-inch rectangle.
3. Roll the dough around the franks leaving the ends open. Put them in the freezer to firm up for about five minutes.
4. Take them out and arrange them in the fryer for 6-8 minutes. Adjust the temperature to 390° Fahrenheit and continue to cook for approximately three minutes.

Sausage & Cheese Wraps

Yields Provided: 8 wraps
Ingredients:
- Crescent roll dough (1 8-count can)
- American cheese (2 slices)
- Heat & Serve Sausages (8)
- Wooden skewers (8)
- _For Dipping_: Ketchup, BBQ sauce or syrup

Preparation Technique:
1. Open the sausages and separate the rolls. Slice the cheese into quarters.
2. Place the franks in paper towels to drain before preparation. Add the cheese strips starting on the widest part of the triangle to the tip. Add the sausage.
3. Pull up each of the ends of the wrap to roll over the sausage and cheese. Be sure to pinch each of the sides together; adding these in two batches to the Air Fryer.
4. Set the fryer temperature at 380° Fahrenheit. Cook for 3-4 minutes depending on how crispy you like the bread.
5. Remove from the fryer and add it to a skewer. Set it out for serving with the desired garnishes.

Spring Rolls

Yields Provided: 20 Servings
Ingredients:
- Noodles (.33 cup)
- Hot water (2 tbsp.)
- Mixed vegetables (1 cup)
- Ground beef (1 cup)
- Spring rolls (1 pkg.)
- Minced garlic cloves (3)
- Small diced onion (1)
- Soy sauce (as desired)
- *Also Needed:* 1 skillet
- For Brushing: Olive oil

Preparation Technique:
1. Dump the noodles into hot water to soften. Drain and slice into short segments.
2. Warm the Air Fryer in advance to 350° Fahrenheit.
3. Heat the skillet (med. heat) and add a spritz the cooking oil spray. Toss in the garlic, onion, ground beef, and mixed veggies. If you have a keto-friendly soy sauce (liquid aminos), add that and sauté for three minutes or until lightly browned.
4. Place on the countertop and add the prepared noodles. Stir and set aside for now.
5. Starting diagonally, add the stuffing to the egg roll. Fold the sheet starting at the top, then the sides, and brush the final side with the water before rolling the wrap closed.
6. Brush the rolls with oil and arrange it in the fryer. Cook for eight minutes and serve.

Taco Fried Egg Rolls

Yields Provided: 8 Servings
Ingredients:
- Lean 93% ground beef (1 lb.)
- Onion (.5 of 1)
- Egg roll wrappers (16)
- Cilantro Lime Rotel (1o oz. can)
- Taco seasoning (half of 1 pkg.)
- Fat-free refried black beans (.5 of 1 can)
- Olive oil (1 tbsp.)
- Reduced-fat Mexican cheese (1 cup)
- Frozen whole kernel corn (.5 cup)

Preparation Technique:
1. Set the fryer temperature to reach 400° Fahrenheit.
2. Dice the onion and garlic. Prepare a frying pan using the med-high heat setting to sauté the garlic and onions.
3. Toss in the beef, salt, pepper, and seasoning pack. Blend in the corn, beans, and Rotel.
4. Prepare the wrappers on a flat surface. Glaze the wrappers with a brush dipped in water along the edges to make the roll easier to close.
5. Load them using two wrappers. Sprinkle each one with cheese. Roll them up and tuck in each end. Spray with a spritz of olive oil.
6. Add to the fryer and set the timer for eight minutes. Flip the rolls over and cook for another four minutes. The time may vary – depending on the size of the cooker.
7. _Note:_ You don't need to double wrap, but it will be a bit messy.

Zucchini Roll-Ups

Yields Provided: 2 Servings
Ingredients:
- Goat cheese (1 cup)
- Zucchini (3)
- Sea salt (as desired)
- Black pepper (.25 tsp.)
- Olive oil (1 tbsp.)

Preparation Technique:
1. Set the Air Fryer at 390° Fahrenheit.
2. Thinly slice the zucchini - lengthwise. Brush each strip using the oil.
3. Mix the cheese, salt, and pepper. Scoop onto the zucchini strips, roll, and securely close using a toothpick.
4. Arrange in the fryer and set the timer for 5 minutes.

Salty Snacks

Cajun Spiced Snack Mix

Yields Provided: 10 cups
Ingredients - The Mix:
- Cajun or Creole seasoning (2 tbsp.)
- Melted butter (.5 cup)
- Mini pretzels (2 cups)
- Peanuts (2 cups)
- Mini wheat thin crackers (2 cups)
- Plain popcorn (4 cups)

Ingredients - The Seasoning:
- Paprika (1 tsp.)
- Garlic (1 tsp.)
- Cayenne pepper (1 tsp.)
- Black pepper (1 tsp.)
- Salt (2 tsp.)
- Onion powder (.5 tsp.)
- Thyme (.5 tsp.)
- Oregano (.5 tsp.)

Preparation Technique:
1. Heat the Air Fryer in advance to reach 370° Fahrenheit.
2. Mix the Cajun seasoning and melted butter together.
3. Combine the pretzels, crackers, popcorn, and peanuts in a mixing container. Empty the butter over the snack and toss.
4. Prepare two batches. Add half of the fixings into the Air Fryer for eight to ten minutes. Toss during the process for even cooking.
5. Cool on a cookie sheet. Store in an air-tight container.

Cheesy Coconut Balls

Yields Provided: 5 Servings
Ingredients:
- Egg (1)
- Mozzarella balls (8 oz. pkg.)
- Coconut flakes (.5 cup)
- Almond flour (.5 cup)

As Desired:
- Paprika
- Thyme
- Pepper

Preparation Technique:
1. Set the Air Fryer temperature to 400° Fahrenheit.
2. Whisk the egg in one bowl and combine the spices with flour in a separate bowl.
3. Sprinkle the balls with the coconut flakes and the flour.
4. Freeze the cheese balls for about 5 minutes. Remove add to the Air Fryer to cook for three minutes and serve.

Chicken Cracklings

Yields Provided: 4 Servings
Ingredients:
- Chicken skins (8)
- Kosher salt (.5 tsp.)

Preparation Technique:
1. Pat each of the chicken skins until dry using a paper towel, adding a sprinkle of salt on both sides.
2. Lay three or four chicken skins in a single layer, skin-side down, on the Air Fryer basket. Set the temperature at 400° Fahrenheit for a total of 12 minutes.
3. At the halfway point (6 min.), flip the chicken skins over - skin-side up.
4. Air fry the chicken skins 6 minutes more or until crispy. Add a minute or two to the cooking time if the skin is still a little flabby in parts.
5. Remove the cracklings from the fryer and place on a wire rack to cool.
6. Dump out any chicken fat on the bottom of the Air Fryer before repeating the steps with the remaining chicken skins.
7. *Note*: Thighs are excellent for the skin choice.

Chickpeas with Ranch Seasoning

Yields Provided: 4 Servings5
Ingredients:
- Lemon juice (2 tbsp.)
- Chickpeas (15 oz. can)
- Olive oil – divided (2 tbsp.)
- Sea salt (1 tsp.)
- Ranch seasoning (1 pkg.)

Preparation Technique:
1. Set then Air Fryer at 400° Fahrenheit.
2. Squeeze the lemon and set the juice aside for now. Drain - don't rinse - the chickpeas and add them to a bowl with one tablespoon of oil. Air fry for 15 minutes.
3. Toss the chickpeas back into the dish and toss in the remainder of the oil, salt, seasoning, and lemon juice.
4. Lower the temperature setting to 350° Fahrenheit.
5. Add the chickpeas back into the fryer at for another five minutes
6. Serve. They'll be good if stored on the countertop for a couple of days.

Corn Tortilla Chips

Yields Provided: 1 Serving
Ingredients:
- Corn tortillas (8)
- Olive oil (1 tbsp.)
- Salt (as desired)

Preparation Technique:
1. Program the Air Fryer temperature setting in advance to 392° Fahrenheit.
2. Use a sharp knife to cut the tortillas, and brush each tortilla with oil.
3. Air fry two batches for three minutes each. Sprinkle with a pinch of salt.

Feta Triangles

Yields Provided: 4 Servings
Ingredients:
- Feta cheese (4 oz.)
- Egg yolk (1)
- Flat-leafed parsley (2 tbsp.)
- Phyllo pastry (2 sheets)
- Olive oil (2 tbsp.)
- Ground black pepper (as desired)
- Finely chopped scallion (1)

Preparation Technique:
1. Finely chop the parsley.
2. Set the temperature setting on the Air Fryer to 390° Fahrenheit.
3. Whisk the egg, scallion, feta, and parsley.
4. Slice the dough into three strips, and a heaping teaspoon of the feta mix underneath the pastry strip.
5. Fold the tip to form a triangle as you work your way around the strip.
6. Use a small amount of oil and brush each triangle before placing them in the cooker basket cooking. Fry for three minutes.
7. Reduce the temperature setting to 360° Fahrenheit, and continue cooking for another two minutes.

Fried Pickles

Yields Provided: 14 pickles

Ingredients:
- All-purpose flour (.25 cup)
- Baking powder (.125 tsp.)
- Dill pickles (14 - refrigerated & crunchy)
- Salt (1 pinch)
- Dark beer (3 tbsp.)
- Water (2-3 tbsp.)
- Panko breadcrumbs (6 tbsp.)
- Cornstarch (2 tbsp.)
- Cayenne pepper (1 pinch)
- Paprika (.5 tsp.)
- *For Frying*: Organic canola or oil spray
- Ranch dressing (.25 to .5 cup)

Preparation Technique:
1. Use paper towels to dry the pickles. Set aside for later.
2. Mix the beer, two tablespoons of water, salt, baking powder, and flour. Its consistency should be similar to regular waffle batter.
3. Prepare two platters. One will have the cornstarch, and the other will have a pinch of salt, the cayenne, paprika, and breadcrumbs.
4. Thinly slice and bread the pickles. Prepare the working surface with the pickles, cornstarch, beer batter, and panko mixture.
5. Dip each of the pickles into the cornstarch and remove excess starch. Dip each one into the batter until evenly covered. Let the excess batter drip away. Lastly, add the pickle into the panko mixture to adequately cover all surfaces.
6. Add the finished pickles to the air fryer basket. Heat the fryer to 360° Fahrenheit.
7. Do this in batches, spraying each layer using a spritz of

cooking oil. Check the pickles after eight minutes. If not ready, add them back and continue cooking checking every minute.

8. Serve with the ranch dressing and enjoy.

Garlic - Roasted Almonds

Yields Provided: 8 Servings

Ingredients:
- Paprika (.25 tsp.)
- Garlic powder (1 tbsp.)
- Raw almonds (2 cups)
- Soy sauce (1 tbsp.)

Preparation Technique:
1. Warm the Air Fryer prior to the baking time to reach 320° Fahrenheit.
2. Stir everything together, omitting the almonds for now to form a thick paste.
3. Now, fold in the almonds. Toss well to coat and place them into the fryer basket to cook for 6-8 minutes.
4. Check every 2-3 minutes to prevent the almonds from sticking. After about six minutes, check every minute. They're done when the inside is also crunchy.
5. Cool for 10-15 minutes. They will remain delicious for 2-3 days.

Kale Chips

Yields Provided: 2 Servings
Ingredients:
- Cabbage (1 head)
- Olive oil (1 tbsp.)
- Soy sauce (1 tsp.)

Preparation Technique:
1. Rinse the kale and dry. Toss into a mixing bowl with the remainder of the fixings.
2. Set the fryer at 200° Fahrenheit and add the kale. Toss halfway through the cycle. Serve.

Onion & Cheese Nuggets

Yields Provided: 4 Servings

Ingredients:
- Egg (1)
- Diced spring onions (2)
- Salt and pepper (to your liking)
- Dried thyme (1 tbsp.)
- Coconut oil (1 tbsp.)
- Grated Edam cheese (7 oz.)

Preparation Technique:
1. Heat the Air Fryer to 350° Fahrenheit
2. Combine each of the fixings (omitting the cheese for now).
3. Make eight balls out of the mixture and stuff the cheese in the center. Store in the refrigerator for one hour.
4. Whisk the egg using a pastry brush to coat the nuggets.
5. Pour them into the Air Fryer for 12 minutes.
6. Serve.

Onion Pakora

Yields Provided: 6 Servings
Ingredients:
- Rice flour (.25 cup)
- Graham flour (1 cup)
- Olive oil (2 tsp.)
- Salt (as desired)
- Carom seed powder (.25 tsp.)
- Turmeric powder (.25 tsp.)
- Freshly chopped coriander (1 tbsp.)
- Green chili peppers (2 finely diced)
- Olive oil (2 tsp.)
- Chili powder (.125 tsp.)

Preparation Technique:
1. Heat the Air Fryer in advance to 350° Fahrenheit.
2. Combine the rice, graham flour and oil. Add small amounts of water as needed to reach the desired consistency.
3. Blend in the peppers, carom, coriander, onions, turmeric, and chili powder.
4. Roll the mixture into small balls and arrange them in the fryer.
5. Set the timer for eight minutes and serve using a splash of hot sauce or other spices you may like.

Roasted Cashews

Yields Provided: 5 Servings
Ingredients:
- Salt (.5 tsp.)
- Coriander powder (1 tsp.)
- Black pepper (.5 tsp.)
- Red chili powder (1 tsp.)
- Cashews (1.66 cups)
- Olive oil (1 tsp.)

Preparation Technique:
1. Preheat the Air Fryer at 250° Fahrenheit.
2. Combine each of the fixings in a mixing container.
3. Toss well and add to the fryer basket. Fry until lightly browned (10 min.).

Spiced Nuts

Yields Provided: 3 cups
Ingredients:
- Egg white (1)
- Ground cloves (.25 tsp.)
- Cinnamon (.5 tsp.)
- Cayenne pepper (1 pinch)
- Salt (as desired)
- Almonds (1 cup)
- Pecan halves (1 cup)
- Cashews (1 cup)

Preparation Technique:
1. Mix the spices with the egg white.
2. Warm up the fryer to 250° Fahrenheit.
3. Toss the nuts into the mixture and shake.
4. Set the timer for the Air Fryer for 25 minutes; stirring several times.
5. Serve after cooling slightly.

Sweet Potato Chips

Yields Provided: 2 Servings

Ingredients:

- Large sweet potatoes (2)
- Salt (as desired)
- Olive oil (2 tbsp.)
- *Also Needed*: Mandoline slicer

Preparation Technique:

1. Warm up the Air Fryer (350° Fahrenheit.).
2. Slice the potatoes with the mandoline and add to a large bowl. Add the oil and toss to coat.
3. Place the chips in the fryer for about 15 minutes or until they're crispy.

Sweet Snacks

Chocolate Chip Cookies

Yields Provided: 5 Servings
Ingredients:

- Egg (1)
- Almond flour (1 cup)
- Dark chocolate chips (2 tbsp.)
- Unsalted butter (3 tbsp.)
- Crushed macadamia nuts (3 tbsp.)
- Vanilla extract (.5 tsp.)
- Stevia (1 tsp.)
- Bak. powder (.25 tsp.)
- Salt (.25 tsp.)

Preparation Technique:

1. Whisk the eggs and blend in the butter and flour.
2. Mix in the remainder of the fixings. Knead the dough.
3. Make five balls for the cookie dough.
4. Set the Air Fryer to 360° Fahrenheit to warm for a minute.
5. Arrange the cookies in the fryer and flatten (just a little). Set the timer for 15 minutes.
6. Cool slightly and serve.

Coconut Chips

Yields Provided: 2 Servings

Ingredients:

- Shredded coconut – large pieces (2 cups)
- Chili powder (1 tbsp.)
- Liquid stevia (.33 tsp.)

Preparation Technique:

1. Warm the Air Fryer to reach 390° Fahrenheit.
2. Mix each of the fixings and toss them into the fryer.
3. Set the timer for five minutes and serve.

Pineapple Sticks with Yogurt Dip

Yields Provided: 2 Servings
Ingredients:

- Pineapple (half of 1)
- Dried coconut (.25 cup)
- Vanilla yogurt (1 cup)
- Fresh mint (1 sprig)

Preparation Technique:

1. Warm up the fryer to 390° Fahrenheit.
2. Slice the pineapple into sticks and dip in the coconut.
3. Arrange in the Air Fryer basket. Set a timer for 10 minutes.
4. Prepare the dip and dice the mint leaves. Combine and serve.

Red Apple Chips

Yields Provided: 6-8 Servings
Ingredients:
- Large red apples (6)
- Olive oil (1 tbsp.)
- Cinnamon (1 pinch)

Preparation Technique:
1. Warm the Air Fryer in advance to 356° Fahrenheit.
2. Slice the apple lengthwise and add them into the Air Fryer basket with a teaspoon of oil.
3. Cook until they're crunchy (10 min.).
4. Sprinkle using the cinnamon, toss, and serve.

Rolled Cookies

Yields Provided: 8 Servings

Ingredients:
- Liquid stevia (4 tbsp.)
- Softened butter (1.5 cups)
- Large eggs (4)
- Almond flour (4 cups)
- Bak. powder (2 tbsp.)
- Salt (1 tsp.)
- Vanilla extract (1 tbsp.)

Preparation Technique:
1. Cream the stevia with the butter in a deep mixing dish.
2. Fold in the vanilla and eggs. Mix in the baking powder, salt, and flour. Cover the batter. Store in the fridge for two hours to chill.
3. Warm the Air Fryer to reach 390° Fahrenheit.
4. Roll the dough out using a floured cutting board. Use a cookie cutter to make the cookie shapes.
5. Arrange the shapes into the fryer basket and bake for 10 minutes or until browned.

Sweet Bacon Peanut Butter Cookies

Yields Provided: 6 Servings
Ingredients:
- Peanut butter (5 tbsp.)
- Bacon (4 slices)
- Swerve (3 tbsp.)
- Ground ginger (.25 tsp.)
- Baking soda (.25 tsp.)
- Vanilla extract (.5 tsp.)

Preparation Technique:
1. Warm up the Air Fryer to 350° Fahrenheit. Prepare the bacon and set aside to drain.
2. Combine all of the fixings – bacon last – in a large mixing container.
3. Shape it into a log. Break it apart into six segments. Roll the balls and gently flatten.
4. Arrange the cookies in the fryer basket and air-fry for 7 minutes.
5. Chill when done and enjoy.

Chapter 12: Desserts

Air Fried Plantains

Yields Provided: 4 Servings
Ingredients:
- Avocado or sunflower oil (2 tsp.)
- Ripened – almost brown – plantains (2)
- *Optional*: Salt (.125 tsp.)

Preparation Technique:
1. Warm up the Air Fryer to 400° Fahrenheit.
2. Slice the plantains at an angle for a .5-inch thickness.
3. Mix the oil, salt, and plantains in a container – making sure you coat the surface thoroughly.
4. Set the timer for eight to ten minutes; shake after five minutes. If they are not done to your liking; add a minute or two more.

Apricot & Blackberry Crumble

Yields Provided: 6 Servings
Ingredients:
- Fresh blackberries (5.5 oz.)
- Lemon juice (2 tbsp.)
- Fresh apricots (18 oz.)
- Sugar (.5 cup)
- Salt (1 pinch)
- Flour (1 cup)
- Cold butter (5 tbsp.)

Preparation Technique:
1. Heat the Air Fryer to 390° Fahrenheit.
2. Lightly grease an 8-inch oven dish with a spritz of cooking oil.
3. Remove the stones, cut the apricots into cubes, and put them in a container.
4. Combine the lemon juice, blackberries, and two tablespoons of sugar with the apricots and mix. Place the fruit in the oven dish.
5. Combine the salt, remainder of the sugar, and flour in a mixing container. Add one tablespoon of cold water and the butter; using your fingertips to make a crumbly mixture.
6. Sprinkle the crumble mixture over the fruit, and press them down.
7. Place the dish in the basket and slide it into the Air Fryer. Fry for 20 minutes. It is ready when it is cooked thoroughly, and the top is browned.

Blackberry Pie

Yields Provided: 8 Servings
Ingredients:
- Stevia (1 scoop)
- Large egg (1)
- Unsalted butter (2 tbsp.)
- Baking powder (1 tbsp.)
- Almond flour (1 cup)
- Blackberries (.5 cup)

Preparation Technique:
1. Warm the Air Fryer to reach 350° Fahrenheit.
2. Whisk the egg and mix with the butter, stevia, and baking powder.
3. Reserve 1 teaspoon of flour, and add the remainder to the mixture. Knead until smooth – not sticky.
4. Cover the fryer basket with the paper and add the dough. Flatten into the shape of a pie crust and add the berries. Sprinkle with the rest of the almond flour on top.
5. Air fry until it's golden (20 min.) Chill before slicing to serve.

Blueberry Hand Pies

Yields Provided: 8 Servings

Ingredients:
- Refrigerated pie crust (14 oz.)
- Blueberries (1 cup)
- Castor sugar (2.5 tbsp.)
- Lemon juice (1 tsp.)
- Salt (1 pinch)
- Water
- *Optional*: Vanilla sugar

Preparation Technique:
1. Mix the sugar, lemon juice, salt, and blueberries, in a medium mixing container.
2. Roll out the pie crusts and cut out six to eight 4--inch individual circles.
3. Scoop about 1 tablespoon of the blueberry filling in the center of each circle.
4. Moisten the edges of dough with a little water. Fold the dough over the filling to form a half-moon shape.
5. Using a fork, gently crimp the edges of the crust together. Then slice three slits on the top of the hand pies.
6. Spray the hand pies with a spritz of cooking oil spray. Sprinkle with vanilla sugar if using.
7. Heat the Air Fryer to reach 350° Fahrenheit.
8. Place three to four hand pies in a single layer inside the Air Fryer basket.
9. Cook for 9 to 12 minutes or until golden brown.
10. Let each of the hand pies cool for at least 10 minutes before serving.

Buttery Lemon Cake

Yields Provided: 16 Servings

Ingredients:

- Warmed butter (2 cups)
- Liquid stevia (.25 cups)
- Sea salt (1 pinch)
- Large eggs (4)
- Baking powder (2 tbsp.)
- Almond flour (2 cups)
- Grated lemon rind (1)

Preparation Technique:

1. Set the Air Fryer temperature at 320° Fahrenheit.
2. Use a layer of parchment paper or use a coating of butter to line a baking tin.
3. Heat two cups of butter with the salt and stevia.
4. Zest the lemon and combine with the eggs, mixing until creamy.
5. Sift in the baking powder and flour. Empty the batter into the baking pan.
6. Set the timer for 35 minutes. Cool slightly and serve.

Caramel Cream-Dipped Apple Fries

Yields Provided: 8-10 Servings

Ingredients:

- Honey-crisp apples/your choice (3)
- Graham cracker crumbs (1 cup)
- Eggs (3)
- Flour (.5 cup)
- Sugar (.25 cup)
- Whipped cream cheese (8 oz.)
- Caramel sauce (.5 cup + more for garnish)

Preparation Technique:

1. Peel and slice the apples into eight wedges. Toss the flour and apple slices together.
2. Prepare a dish with the eggs. Mix the sugar and crackers in another bowl. Dip the apples in the eggs, and then the crumb mixture coating all sides. Arrange on a baking tray.
3. Set the fryer to 380° Fahrenheit. Brush or spray the bottom of the fryer with a spritz of oil.
4. Prepare in two batches. Start by placing them in a single layer –spraying each batch lightly. Cook for five minutes, flip, and cook for another two minutes.
5. Make the cream dip by combining the caramel sauce and cream cheese.
6. Serve the hot apple fries with the caramel dip.

Cheesecake with Sliced Almonds

Yields Provided: 6 Servings
Ingredients:
- Almonds (.5 cup)
- Soft butter (6 tbsp.)
- Stevia (1 tbsp.)
- Vanilla extract (.5 tsp.)
- Cream cheese (1 cup)
- Eggs (2)
- Swerve (2 tbsp.)
- Cinnamon (.25 tsp.)
- Lemon zest (1 tsp.)

Preparation Technique:
1. Combine the butter, vanilla, stevia, and sliced almonds.
2. Cover the Air Fryer tray with the paper and add the cheesecake crust (step 1). Combine the cinnamon, swerve, lemon zest, and cream cheese.
3. Use a hand mixer to prepare the eggs until fluffy. Pour the cream cheese mixture over the almond crust.
4. Set the Air Fryer temperature to 310° Fahrenheit. Set the timer for 16 minutes. When done, chill for at least two hours.
5. Slice and serve.

Chocolate Cake

Yields Provided: 4 Servings
Ingredients:
- Unchilled butter (1 stick)
- Cocoa powder (.33 cup)
- Baking powder (1 tsp.)
- Baking soda (.5 tsp.)
- Eggs (3)
- Sour cream (.5 cup)
- Flour (1 cup)
- Sugar (.66 cup)
- Vanilla (2 tsp.)

Preparation Technique:
1. Set the Air Fryer to 320° Fahrenheit.
2. Mix ingredients on using the low setting of an electric mixer.
3. Pour into the oven attachment. Pour it into the basket and slide it into the Air Fryer.
4. Set the timer to 25 minutes. Once the timer buzzes, lightly push in the center to see if the cake is done. If it does not spring back when touched, cook for an additional 5 minutes.
5. Cool the cake on a wire rack. Ice with your favorite frosting.

Chocolate Soufflés

Yields Provided: 2 Servings
Ingredients:
- Semi-sweet chocolate (3 oz. - chopped)
- Butter (.25 cup)
- Eggs (2 separated)
- Sugar (3 tbsp.)
- All-purpose flour (2 tbsp.)
- Pure vanilla extract (.5 tsp.)
- *Optional*: Whipped cream for topping
- Powdered sugar for garnish
- *Also Needed*: Two 6-oz. ramekins

Preparation Technique:
1. Spread butter and sugar in the ramekins; shake, and dump out the excess of sugar.
2. Melt the butter and chocolate in a double boiler or microwave.
3. Whisk the egg yolks. Blend in the sugar and vanilla, stir and add the butter/chocolate mixture. Lastly, add the flour and mix until the lumps are gone.
4. Heat the fryer to reach 330° Fahrenheit.
5. Whisk the egg whites to form soft peaks and slowly fold into the chocolate mixture.
6. Pour the prepared batter in the greased/sugared ramekins. Leave a ½-inch space at the top. Arrange them in the basket of the fryer and air-fry for 14 minutes until browned on the top.
7. Dust using the sugar and serve. You can also pour some heavy cream over the soufflé at the table.

Donut Bread Pudding

Yields Provided: 4 Servings

Ingredients:

- Glazed donuts (6)
- Raw egg yolks (4)
- Whipping cream (1.5 cups)
- Sugar (.25 cups)
- Frozen sweet cherries (.75 cups)
- Cinnamon (1 tsp.)
- Semi-sweet chocolate baking chips (.5 cup)
- Raisins (.5 cup)

Preparation Technique:

1. Preheat the fryer at 310° Fahrenheit.
2. Toss the wet fixings in a container and add everything else.
3. Pour into a baking pan and cover it with foil. Place it into the basket and set the timer for one hour.
4. Chill the pudding thoroughly before serving.

Fried Banana Smores

Yields Provided: 4 Servings
Ingredients:
- Bananas (4)
- Mini-peanut butter chips (3 tbsp.)
- Graham cracker cereal (3 tbsp.)
- Mini-semi-sweet chocolate chips (3 tbsp.)

Preparation Technique:
1. Heat the Air Fryer in advance to 400° Fahrenheit.
2. Slice the un-peeled bananas lengthwise along the inside of the curve. *Don't slice through the bottom of the peel.* Open slightly - forming a pocket.
3. Fill each pocket with chocolate chips, peanut butter chips, and marshmallows. Poke the cereal into the filling.
4. Arrange the stuffed bananas in the fryer basket, keeping them upright with the filling facing up.
5. Air-fry until the peel has blackened and the chocolate and marshmallows have toasted (6 min.).
6. Cool for a couple of minutes. Spoon out the filling to serve.

Green Avocado Pudding

Yields Provided: 3 Servings

Ingredients:

- Pitted avocado (1)
- Almond milk (5 tbsp.)
- Stevia (3 tsp.)
- Vanilla extract (.25 tsp.)
- Salt (.25 tsp.)
- Cocoa powder (1 tbsp.)

Preparation Technique:

1. Heat the Air Fryer for 2-3 minutes at 360° Fahrenheit.
2. Peel and mash the avocado and mix with the milk, salt, vanilla extract, stevia, and cocoa powder.
3. Prepare in the Air Fryer for three minutes.
4. Chill thoroughly and serve.

Holiday Cherry Pie

Yields Provide 8 Servings
Ingredients:
- Refri d pie crusts (2)
- Ch filling (21 oz. can)
- M p.)
- F 1)

Prepar chnique:
1. the fryer to 310° Fahrenheit.
2. Poke holes into the crust after placing it in a pie plate. Allow the excess to hang over the edges. Place in the Air Fryer for five minutes
3. Transfer the basket with the pie plate onto the countertop. Fill it with the cherries. Remove the excess crust.
4. Cut the remaining crust into ¾-inch strips placing weaving a lattice across the pie.
5. Make an egg wash with milk and egg. Brush the pie. Bake for 15minutes. Serve with an ice cream of your choice.

Lemon Ricotta Cheesecake

Yields Provided: 4 Servings
Ingredients:
- Defrosted sheets filo pastry/homemade (4)
- Melted butter (2 oz.)
- Chunky peanut butter (4 tbsp.)
- Marshmallow fluff (4 tsp.)
- Sea salt (1 pinch)

Preparation Technique:
1. Set the temperature of the Air Fryer at 360° Fahrenheit.
2. Use melted butter to brush a sheet of filo. Put the second sheet on top and brush it also. Continue the process until you've completed all four sheets. Cut the layers into four (4) 12-inch by 3-inch strips.
3. Place one teaspoon of the marshmallow fluff on the underside and one tablespoon of peanut butter. Fold the tip over the filo strip to form a triangle, making sure the filling is completely wrapped.
4. Seal the ends with a small amount of butter. Place the completed turnovers into the Air Fryer for three to five minutes.
5. When done, they'll be golden brown.
6. Add a touch of sea salt for the sweet/salty challenge.
7. *Special Notes*: The Phyllo/Filo pastry is a little different than regular pastry. It is tissue-thin and has minimal fat content. It is considered acceptable by some bakers and is interchange the filo with regular puff pastry for turnovers.

Marshmallow & Yam Hand Pies

Yields Provided: 4 Servings
Ingredients:
- Crescent dough sheet/homemade crust (1)
- Candied yams (16 oz. can)
- Cinnamon (.5 tsp.)
- Allspice (.25 tsp.)
- Salt (.25 tsp.)
- Marshmallow crème (2 tbsp.)
- Egg (1)

Ingredients - The Maple Glaze:
- Confectioners' sugar (.5 cup)
- Maple syrup (.5 cup)

Preparation Technique:
1. Set the temperature on the Air Fryer to 400° Fahrenheit.
2. Drain the syrup from the yams and combine with the cinnamon, salt, and allspice using a fork until fully mixed.
3. Put the dough sheet onto a board and cut it into four equal segments.
4. Spoon the filling onto the squares and add a tablespoon of the crème.
5. Use a brush to spread the egg over the edges of the dough and place the remainder of the two pieces of dough on top of the pies.
6. Use a fork to crimp the edges, and cut three slits in the top for venting.
7. Arrange in the Air Fryer for six minutes.
8. Prepare the glaze using the sugar and syrup in a small

dish—slowly adding the syrup—until the sugar dissolves.

9. To serve, drizzle the glaze over the warm pies and enjoy.

Pumpk[...]

Yields Provi[...]

Ingredients:

- Melted butt[...]
- Large flour to[...]
- Sugar (1 cup)
- Orange sanding su[...]
- Whole milk ricotta (2 [...]
- Ground cinnamon (1 tbs[...]
- Confectioners' sugar (.66 cu[...]
- Pumpkin pie mix (1.5 cups)
- Mini chocolate chips (.5 cup)

Preparation Technique:

1. Let the Air Fryer get hot for three m[...] Fahrenheit.
2. Use a pumpkin cookie cutter to make the tort[...]
3. Brush one side of the cut-outs with the butt[...] scatter them with the orange sanding sugar.
4. Combine the cinnamon and regular sugar in a sma[...] dish. Sprinkle the mixture over the cookies.
5. Bake in batches until crispy (about 3 minutes). Use wire racks for cooling.
6. Make the dip by using a large bowl; combine the cinnamon sugar, pumpkin pie, mix, and ricotta in a large mixing dish. Stir well.
7. Be creative and place the dip in a shallow serving platter.
8. Place the crisps into the dip to make a pumpkin patch and decorate with the chips.

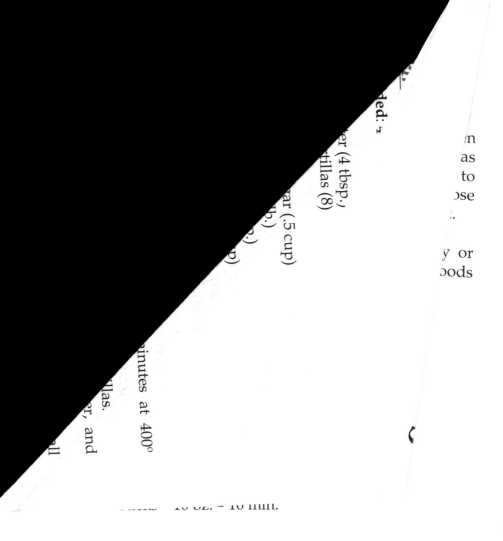

...z. – 10 min.

Steak Options at 400° Fahrenheit:

- London Broil – 2 lb. – 20-28 min.
- Bone-In Rib Eye – 1-inch – 8 oz. – 10-15 min.
- Filet Mignon – 8 oz. – 18 min.
- Flank Steak – 1 ½ lb. – 12 min.
- Sirloin Steaks – 1-inch – 12 oz. – 9-14 min.

Veggie Options at 400° Fahrenheit:

- Small Baby Potatoes – 1 ½ lb. – 15 min.

- Potatoes – 1-inch chunks – 12 min.
- Whole Baked Potatoes – 40 min.
- Squash – ½ inch chunks – 12 min.
- Cherry Tomatoes – 4 min.
- Zucchini – ½ inch sticks – 12 min.
- Asparagus – 1-inch slices – 5 min.
- Beets – whole – 40 min.
- Broccoli – florets – 6 min.
- Cauliflower – florets – 12 min.
- Eggplant – 1 ½-inch cubes – 15 min.
- Green Beans – 5 min.
- Mushrooms - sliced ¼-inch thick – 5 min.
- Pearl Onions – 10 min.
- Peppers – 1-inch chunks – 15 min.

These Veggies are best prepared at 380°F:
- Baked Sweet Potato – 30-35 min.
- Brussels Sprouts in halves – 15 min.
- Carrots – ½-inch slices – 15 min.
- Parsnips - ½-inch chunks – 15 min.

Other Veggies:
- Corn on the Cob – 390°F – 6 min.
- Tomatoes – halved – 350°F – 10 min.

Note: Remember, these are estimated times. Each Air Fryer may vary depending on the variations of a particular recipe.
Just For Fun For The Pooch - Puppy Poppers

Yields Provided: Varied
Ingredients:
- Unsweetened applesauce (.5 cup)
- Peanut butter (1 cup)
- Oats (2 cups)

- Baking powder (1 tsp.)
- Flour (1 cup)

Preparation Technique:
1. Mix the peanut butter and applesauce in a mixing bowl until creamy smooth. Fold in the oats, baking powder, and flour. When smooth, roll out the dough into teaspoon-sized balls.
2. Set the Air Fryer at 350° Fahrenheit.
3. Cover the bucket of the fryer basket with a spritz of oil.
4. Arrange 8-12 of the balls in the basket and cook for eight minutes. Turn halfway through the cycle (6 min.).
5. Continue the process with the batter until all are done. Cool completely before storing it.
6. The poppers will stay fresh for up to two weeks.

CPSIA information can be obtained
at www.ICGtesting.com
Printed in the USA
LVHW051729120221
679115LV00005B/237